NO GALLBLADDER DIET COOKBOOK

200+ QUICK & EASY RECIPES TO SOOTHE YOUR DIGESTIVE SYSTEM AFTER GALLBLADDER REMOVAL SURGERY

28-DAY MEAL PLAN INCLUDED

Audrey Robinson

Table of Contents

INTRODUCTION

Have you undergone gallbladder removal or should have this surgery soon? In these cases it is normal to have some concerns about what you can eat next. To help you gain clarity, in this introductory chapter we present some tips for a model-type diet to follow. You will find that despite being a rather restrictive eating program, the recipes that follow will make it easy, tasty, and even enjoyable. We are confident that by following the wealth of alternatives proposed afterwards your life will quickly return to the way it was before. What are you waiting for? Take note and don't worry. Let's start with the basics, what exactly is the gallbladder?

What Is The Gallbladder?

The gallbladder is a small pear-shaped organ located on the right side of the abdomen beneath the liver. To simplify, one can imagine the gallbladder as a pouch whose function is to accumulate and concentrate bile. The liver produces this substance between meals, accumulated in the gallbladder and released into the duodenum (initial tract of the small intestine). It contributes to the digestion and absorption of fats and other substances from nutrition. Following the removal of the gallbladder, digestion is not impaired. Still, there is a lack of bile collection activity, which passes into the intestines in somewhat larger quantities, causing, in some cases, the emission of liquid stools and more rarely, diarrhea. Usually, this phenomenon occurs in the days following surgery, due to the laxative effect of the bile salts themselves, and resolves within a few weeks.

What Can I Eat If I Don't Have a Gallbladder? - Recommended Foods

What foods can you eat after gallbladder or cholecystectomy? This is the main question, and the truth is that you must begin by eliminating fats or eating very low-fat foods, such as vegetable fats, which are generally better tolerated after a cholecystectomy. If you don't have a gallbladder, you should eat the following foods:

- Herbal teas and teas, such as green tea and chamomile tea
- Low-fat dairy products, whether milk, cheese or yogurt
- Legumes without skin and in moderation
- Rice
- Pasta

- Toasted bread and crackers

- Vegetables, except those that are difficult to digest and flatulent

- Fruits such as berries, apples, pears, peaches, etc.

- Lean meats

- White or lean fish

- The only fatty foods allowed: olive or seed oil, preferably raw or well-boiled, never fried.

Foods banned or not recommended after Gallbladder Removal Surgery

Apart from the foods mentioned above, you should consider the foods you should avoid after gallbladder removal surgery to eliminate them from your diet or, if your doctor suggests, to consume the appropriate amounts of them to avoid harm while benefiting from their nutrients.

- Chocolate

- Whole milk

- Coffee

- Fast food

- Refined carbohydrates

- Hydrogenated fats

- Fatty meats, such as sausages

- Fried and processed foods

- Butter

- Eggs, particularly the yolk

- Oily fish and shellfish

- Hard-skinned legumes

- Spicy and sauces

- Olives

- Flatulent vegetables such as cauliflower, cabbage or artichokes

- Very fatty nuts such as hazelnuts and walnuts

There is a common misconception that you can only eat bland, liquid-like, or soft foods after gallbladder surgery. This is not the case. After gallbladder removal surgery, you may be advised to follow a strict post-op diet plan to help heal your digestive system and prevent further complications.

Just because you've undergone gallbladder removal surgery doesn't mean that your days of eating delicious food are over. There are plenty of tasty and nutritious recipes perfect for post-gallbladder surgery diets. That's where this list of 200+ quick and easy recipes comes in handy!

In addition, this cookbook also includes a 28-day meal plan to help you heal your digestive system and get back on track with your healthy eating habits. The following pages will help you discover what foods are ideal for cleansing your digestive tract after gallbladder surgery and how long they should be included in your diet to quickly promote healing of the organ. So, we hope you enjoy these recipes and that they provide you with the nutrients and energy you need to heal quickly and enjoy a delicious meal.

Breakfast

Buckwheat Pancakes

 Prep Time: 10 minutes   Cooking Time: 10 minutes   Servings: 2

INGREDIENTS

2/3 cup raw buckwheat groats, soaked overnight, rinsed & drained
1 egg
¼ tsp cinnamon
1 tsp stevia
¼ tsp sea salt
½ cup water

DIRECTIONS

1. Transfer the buckwheat to a mixer and add in egg, stevia, cinnamon, salt, and water and mix until very smooth.
2. Grease a nonstick skillet and set over medium heat; pour in about a third cup of the buckwheat batter, spreading to cover the bottom of the skillet.
3. Cook for about 2 minutes over the side or until the pancake is golden brown. Repeat with the remaining batter. Serve right away with a glass of orange juice if desired.

Nutrition: Calories: 166; Fat: 3.5 g; Carbs: 26.4 g; Protein: 7.8 g

Turkey Sweet Potato Breakfast Casserole

 Prep Time: 10 minutes   Cooking Time: 45 minutes   Servings: 6

INGREDIENTS

1 tbsp olive oil
1/2-pound ground turkey
1 large sweet potato, cut into slices
1/2 cup spinach
12 eggs
Salt and pepper, as needed

DIRECTIONS

1. Warm the oven to 350 F. Lightly coat a square baking tray with olive oil and set it aside.
2. In your skillet, set over medium heat, brown ground turkey in olive oil; season well, and remove from heat.
3. Layer the potato slices onto the baking tray and top with raw spinach and ground turkey.
4. In a small bowl, whisk the salt, eggs, and pepper until thoroughly mixed; pour over the mixture to cover completely.
5. Bake within 45 minutes, or until the eggs are cooked through, and the potatoes are soft. Remove and let it set aside to cool slightly before serving.

Nutrition: Calories: 247; Fat: 15.2 g; Carbs: 5.9 g; Protein: 22.1 g

Eggs Baked in Mushrooms

 Prep Time: 10 minutes   Cooking Time: 20 minutes   Servings: 2

INGREDIENTS

4 mushrooms
1 tsp black pepper
4 eggs
3 tbsp nonfat or low-fat cheese
3 tbsp parsley
1 tsp garlic powder
2 tbsp olive oil
1 tsp salt
½ tsp pepper

DIRECTIONS

1. Warm the broiler and line a baking sheet.
2. Season the mushrooms with oil, salt, pepper, and ½ tsp garlic powder. Broil for 5 minutes on each side. Remove from oven, then set to 400 F.
3. Crack an egg into each mushroom. Sprinkle some cheese on top, then bake within 15 minutes.
4. Sprinkle with the remaining seasonings and garnish with parsley, then serve.

Nutrition: Calories: 95, Fat: 4g, Carbs: 5g, Protein: 10g

Artichoke Pancakes

 Prep Time: 10 minutes   Cooking Time: 30 minutes   Servings: 4

INGREDIENTS

1 cup whole wheat flour
¼ tsp baking soda
¼ tsp baking powder
1 cup artichoke
2 eggs
1 cup nonfat milk

DIRECTIONS

1. In your bowl, combine all ingredients and mix well.
2. In a skillet, heat olive oil, pour ¼ of the batter and cook each pancake for 1-2 minutes per side.
3. When ready, remove from heat and serve.

Nutrition: Calories: 50, Fat: 0g, Carbs: 9g, Protein: 3g

Breakfast Overnight Oats

 Prep Time: 10 minutes + chilling time

 Cooking Time: 0 minutes

 Servings: 4

INGREDIENTS

1/2 cup old-fashioned oats
1 tsp chia seeds
1/2 cup vanilla almond milk, unsweetened
1/4 cup fresh blueberries
1/4 banana, chopped
1/4 cup chopped fresh pineapple
1/4 cup nonfat Greek yogurt
1/4 tsp cinnamon
1 tbsp chopped toasted almonds

DIRECTIONS

1. Mix the oats, chia seeds, almond milk, blueberries, banana, pineapple, yogurt, cinnamon, and chopped toasted almonds in a small container. Refrigerate for 24 hours.
2. Remove from the refrigerator and whisk thoroughly before serving.

Nutrition: Calories: 290, Fat: 6g, Carbs: 30g, Protein: 22g

Cassava Crepes

 Prep Time: 10 minutes

 Cooking Time: 15 minutes

 Servings: 4

INGREDIENTS

1 1/3 cups cassava flour
2 egg whites
1 cup nonfat or low-fat milk
2 tsp lemon juice
2 tbsp nonfat or low-fat melted butter
1 tsp stevia
1 pinch salt

DIRECTIONS

1. In a mixing bowl, whisk egg whites, milk, lemon juice, butter, stevia, and sea salt; gradually whisk in cassava flour until well mixed and smooth.
2. Preheat a nonstick pan and spread in about a quarter cup of batter to cover the bottom. Cook within 3 minutes per side or until golden brown.
3. Repeat with the remaining batter. Serve with a cup of tea or a glass of juice.

Nutrition: Calories: 227; Fat: 7.5 g; Carbs: 38.69 g; Protein: 3.65 g

Broccoli Frittata

 Prep Time: 10 minutes   Cooking Time: 20 minutes   Servings: 2

INGREDIENTS

1 cup broccoli
1 tbsp olive oil
½ red onion
2 eggs
¼ tsp salt
2 oz nonfat or low-fat cheese
1 garlic clove
¼ tsp dill

DIRECTIONS

1. In your bowl, whisk eggs with salt and cheese.
2. In a frying pan, heat olive oil and pour the egg mixture. Add remaining ingredients and mix well. Serve and enjoy!

Nutrition: Calories: 200, Carbs: 9g, Fat: 9g, Protein: 14g

Amaranth Porridge

 Prep Time: 10 minutes   Cooking Time: 30 minutes   Servings: 2

INGREDIENTS

½ cup amaranth
1 ½ cups water
¼ cup almond milk
1 tsp stevia
¼ tsp sea salt

DIRECTIONS

1. In a pan, mix water, salt, and amaranth and bring to a boil; cover and simmer for about 30 minutes and then stir in milk and stevia.
2. Cook, stirring, until the porridge is creamy. Serve right away.

Nutrition: Calories: 190; Fat: 3.8 g; Carbs: 27.7 g; Protein: 7.3 g

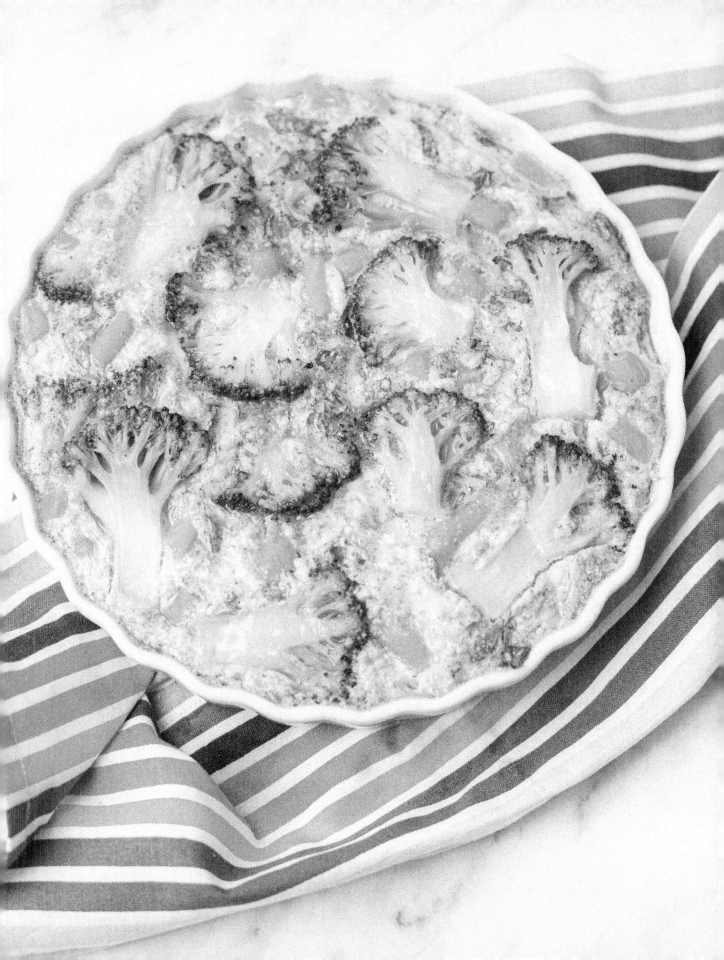

Coconut Yogurt with Acai Berry Granola

 Prep Time: 10 minutes   Cooking Time: 0 minutes   Servings: 2

INGREDIENTS

2 cup unflavored coconut yogurt
2 tsp raw honey
½ cup granola cereal
½ cup frozen acai berries

DIRECTIONS

1. Pour the yogurt into a serving bowl or a glass, stir in raw honey, top with granola, and sprinkle acai berries on top.
2. Serve and enjoy!

Nutrition: Calories: 208, Fat: 7g, Carbs: 12g, Protein: 1g

Greek Omelet

 Prep Time: 5 minutes   Cooking Time: 10 minutes   Servings: 2

INGREDIENTS

3 eggs
½ cup parsley
¼ tsp salt
¼ tsp ground pepper
1 tsp olive oil
¼ cup spinach
1 plum tomato
½ cup nonfat or low-fat feta cheese
6 pitted Kalamata olives

DIRECTIONS

1. In a bowl, whisk together eggs, parsley, pepper, and salt
2. In a skillet, add the egg mixture and sprinkle the remaining ingredients. Cook for 2-3 minutes per side. Serve and enjoy!

Nutrition: Calories: 164, Fat: 4g, Carbs: 14g, Protein: 19g

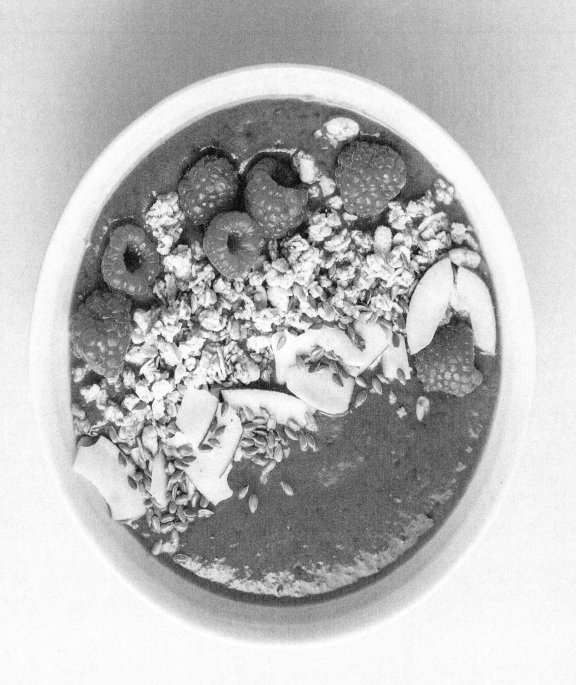

Turmeric Oatmeal

 Prep Time: 5 minutes   Cooking Time: 5 minutes   Servings: 2

INGREDIENTS

2 cups water
1 tsp turmeric powder
Mint leaves, as you like
1 cup whole rolled oats
2 splashes of oat milk

DIRECTIONS

1. Place your rolled oats in a bowl, add turmeric powder, milk, and water and stir to mix.
2. Add toppings, cover, and place in the fridge overnight. Serve in the morning.

Nutrition: Calories: 154, Fat:3.1 g, Carbs:29.2 g, Protein:5.1 g

---

Salmon Egg Salad

 Prep Time: 5 minutes   Cooking Time: 5 minutes   Servings: 2

INGREDIENTS

2 hardboiled eggs
¼ cup red onion
2 tbsp capers
1 tbsp lime juice
3 oz smoked salmon
1 tbsp olive oil

DIRECTIONS

1. In your bowl, combine all ingredients and mix well.
2. Serve with your favorite dressing.

Nutrition: Calories: 237, Fat: 8g, Carbs: 10g, Protein: 37g

Mushroom Omelet

 Prep Time: 5 minutes   Cooking Time: 10 minutes   Servings: 1

INGREDIENTS

2 eggs
¼ tsp salt
¼ tsp black pepper
1 tbsp olive oil
¼ cup nonfat or low-fat cheese
¼ tsp basil
1 cup mushrooms

DIRECTIONS

1. In your bowl, combine all ingredients and mix well
2. In a skillet, heat olive oil, pour the egg mixture, and cook for 1-2 minutes per side
3. Remove the omelet from your skillet and serve!

Nutrition: Calories: 267, Fat: 12g, Carbs: 7g, Protein: 30g

Banana Pancakes

 Prep Time: 10 minutes   Cooking Time: 20 minutes   Servings: 4

INGREDIENTS

1 cup whole wheat flour
¼ tsp baking soda
¼ tsp baking powder
1 cup mashed banana
2 eggs
1 cup nonfat or low-fat milk

DIRECTIONS

1. In your bowl, combine all ingredients and mix well
2. In a skillet, heat olive oil, pour ¼ of the batter and cook each pancake for 1-2 minutes per side. Serve and enjoy!

Nutrition: Calories: 150, Fat: 4g, Carbs: 23g, Protein: 4g

Avocado Toast with Hummus

 Prep Time: 5 minutes   Cooking Time: 0 minutes   Servings: 1

INGREDIENTS

1 slice of toasted whole wheat bread
2 tbsp hummus
1/4 ripe avocado, sliced
A pinch of sea salt
A pinch of black pepper

DIRECTIONS

1. Spread the whole-wheat toast with hummus and top with avocado.
2. Sprinkle with sea salt, plus pepper, and serve.

Nutrition: Calories: 219; Fat: 15.5 g; Carbs: 13.1 g; Protein: 6.8 g

---

Rutabaga Breakfast Hash

 Prep Time: 10 minutes   Cooking Time: 20 minutes   Servings: 2

INGREDIENTS

2 tbsp olive oil
1 rutabaga
¼ cup onion
1 tsp salt
¼ tsp black pepper

DIRECTIONS

1. Heat olive oil and fry rutabaga in a skillet for 3-4 minutes. Cook for another 5-6 minutes or until rutabaga is tender.
2. Add onion, black pepper, and salt and stir to combine. Garnish with dill and serve.

Nutrition: Calories: 95, Carbs: 4g, Fat: 6g, Protein: 6g

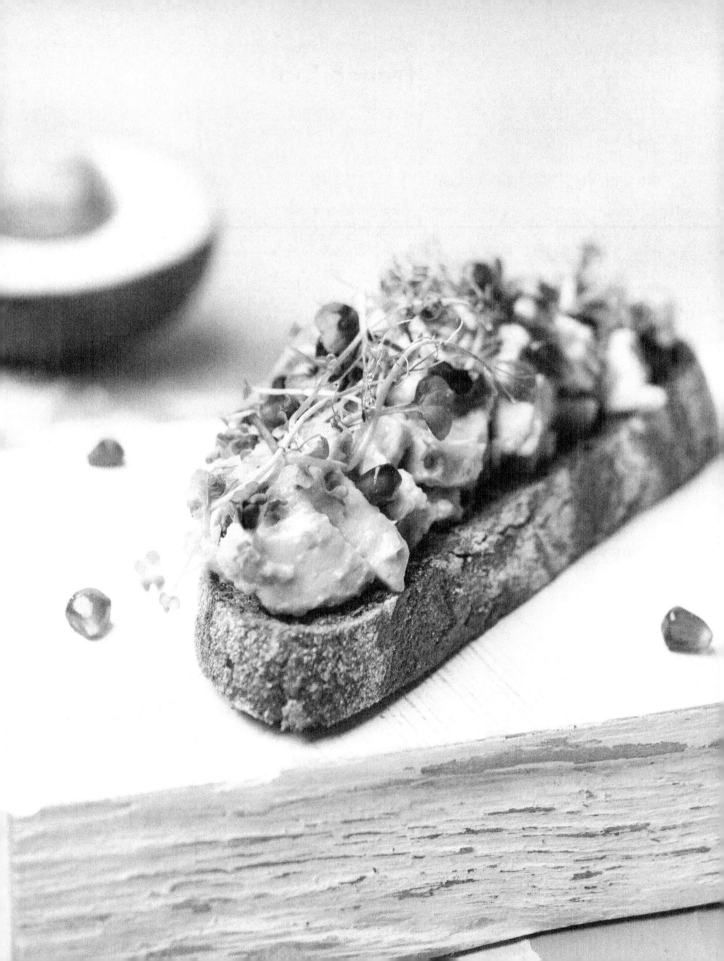

French Toast

 Prep Time: 10 minutes   Cooking Time: 10 minutes   Servings: 2

INGREDIENTS

½ cup peanut butter
2 whole-wheat bread slices
2 eggs
¼ cup almond milk
1 tsp pure vanilla extract
1 tbsp sugar substitute

DIRECTIONS

1. Whisk together eggs, vanilla extract, sugar, and almond milk in a bowl. Spread peanut butter over bread slices and top with bread slices.
2. Dip each sandwich in an egg mixture. Place sandwiches in a pan and cook for 5-6 minutes per side or until golden brown. Serve and enjoy!

Nutrition: Calories: 63, Fat: 1g, Carbs: 9g, Protein: 5g

Mixed Berries Yogurt

 Prep Time: 5 minutes   Cooking Time: 0 minutes   Servings: 1

INGREDIENTS

3 cups nonfat or low-fat Greek yogurt
½ cup almonds
¼ cup blueberries
1 cup strawberries
½ tsp lemon juice

DIRECTIONS

1. In a bowl, place all ingredients, mix well and refrigerate overnight.
2. Serve in the morning.

Nutrition: Calories: 70, Carbs: 17g, Fat: 1g, Protein: 1g

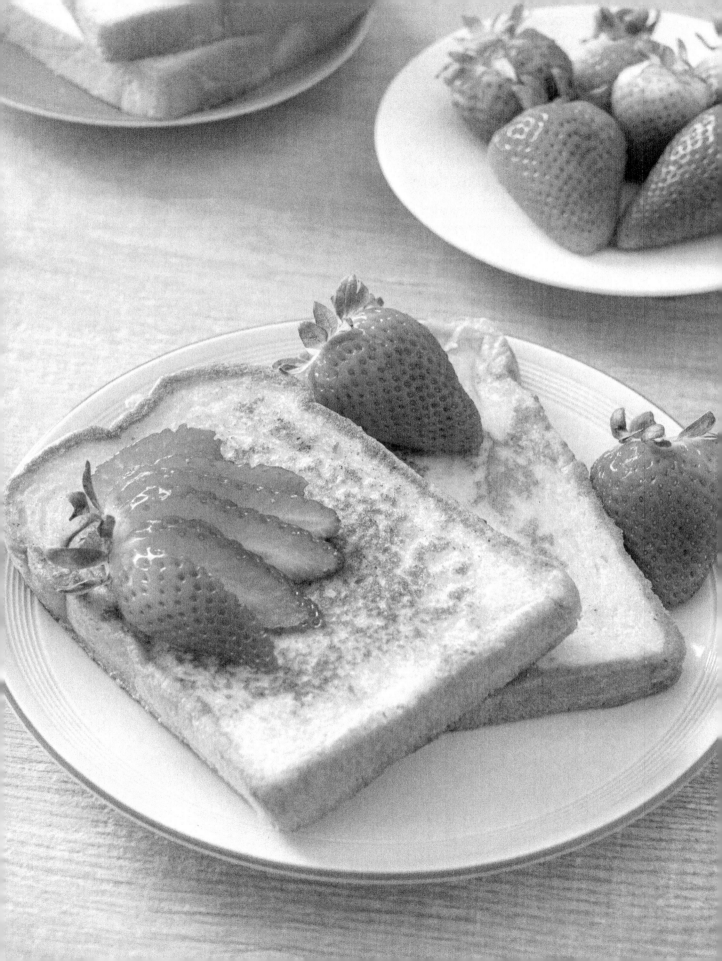

Amaranth with Toasted Walnuts

 Prep Time: 10 minutes   Cooking Time: 25 minutes   Servings: 6

INGREDIENTS

2 cups amaranth
4 cups water
1/2 tsp salt
1 cup chopped toasted walnuts

DIRECTIONS

1. In a pan, mix the amaranth, salt, and water and bring to a boil; cover and simmer within 25 minutes or until liquid is absorbed; remove from heat and let cool for about 5 minutes.
2. Serve the amaranth topped with toasted walnuts.

Nutrition: Calories: 311; Fat: 15.5 g; Carbs: 29.3 g; Protein: 12.1 g

---

Kale Frittata

 Prep Time: 10 minutes   Cooking Time: 20 minutes   Servings: 2

INGREDIENTS

1 cup kale
1 tbsp olive oil
½ red onion
¼ tsp salt
2 oz nonfat or low-fat cheddar cheese
1 garlic clove
2 eggs
¼ tsp dill

DIRECTIONS

1. In your bowl, whisk eggs with salt and cheese until well blended.
2. In a frying pan, heat olive oil and pour the egg mixture. Add remaining ingredients and mix well. Serve and enjoy!

Nutrition: Calories: 195, Fat: 14g, Carbs: 5g, Protein: 14g

Banana And Apple Pancakes

 Prep Time: 5 minutes

 Cooking Time: 5 minutes

 Servings: 3

INGREDIENTS

1 apple
5 eggs
2 bananas
1 tbsp olive oil

DIRECTIONS

1. In a bowl, mash the bananas and apples. Crack the eggs and mix them all.
2. In a frying pan, pour one-two spoon of the mixture, and cook each pancake for 1-2 minutes per side. Remove and serve!

Nutrition: Calories: 338, Fat: 13g, Carbs: 48g, Protein: 9g

Brown Rice Breakfast Bowl

 Prep Time: 10 minutes

 Cooking Time: 10 minutes

 Servings: 4

INGREDIENTS

2 cups cooked brown rice
1/2 cup unsweetened almond milk
1 tsp liquid stevia
1 tbsp almond butter
1 apple, diced
2 dates, chopped
1/2 tsp cinnamon

DIRECTIONS

1. Mix almond oil, almond butter, stevia, apple, and dates in a saucepan; bring to a gentle boil.
2. Cook within 5 minutes or until the apples are tender; stir in cinnamon and brown rice, cook within 5 minutes, and then remove from heat. Serve immediately.

Nutrition: Calories: 226; Fat: 4.3 g; Carbs: 34.4 g; Protein: 5.8 g

Orange Muffins

 Prep Time: 10 minutes

 Cooking Time: 20 minutes

 Servings: 6

INGREDIENTS

1 cup whole wheat flour
½ tbsp granulated stevia
1 tsp baking powder
¼ tsp salt
2 eggs
¼ cup almond milk
½ cup dairy-free butter
1 tsp grated orange rind

DIRECTIONS

1. Preheat the oven to 375 F.
2. Mix flour, stevia, salt, and baking powder in a bowl. Stir together almond, butter, eggs, and dry ingredients and mix well.
3. Spoon batter into your muffin cups, then bake it for 18-20 minutes until golden brown, remove and serve.

Nutrition: Calories: 114, Fat: 1g, Carbs: 25g, Protein: 3g

Nutmeg Apple Frozen Yogurt

 Prep Time: 5 minutes

 Cooking Time: 0 minutes

 Servings: 4

INGREDIENTS

2 apples halves
1 cup nonfat or low-fat Greek yogurt
½ cup coconut sugar
¼ tsp ground nutmeg
⅛ tsp ground cinnamon

DIRECTIONS

1. Puree the apple in a mixer.
2. Mix apple, Greek yogurt, coconut sugar, cinnamon, and nutmeg in an ice cream jar. Freeze for two or more hours before serving.

Nutrition: Calories: 91; Fat: 1.1g; Carbs: 15.5g; Protein: 5.2g

Leek Frittata

 Prep Time: 10 minutes   Cooking Time: 20 minutes   Servings: 2

INGREDIENTS

½ cup leek
1 tbsp olive oil
½ red onion
2 eggs
¼ tsp salt
2 oz nonfat or low-fat parmesan cheese
1 garlic clove
¼ tsp dill

DIRECTIONS

1. In your bowl, whisk eggs with salt and cheese.
2. In a frying pan, heat olive oil and pour the egg mixture. Add remaining ingredients and mix well. Serve and enjoy!

Nutrition: Calories: 162, Fat: 8g, Carbs: 9g, Protein: 11g

Banana Walnut Pancakes

 Prep Time: 10 minutes   Cooking Time: 5 minutes   Servings: 2

INGREDIENTS

1 large banana
2 medium eggs, beaten
pinch of baking powder
splash of pure vanilla extract
1 tsp olive oil
¼ cup walnuts, roughly chopped
½ cup blueberry

DIRECTIONS

1. Mash banana with a fork in your bowl. Add 2 beaten eggs, a pinch of baking powder, and a pinch of vanilla extract.
2. Heat a large nonstick skillet or pancake over medium heat and brush with ½ tsp of oil.
3. With half the batter, pour two pancakes into the pan, cook 1 to 2 minutes per side, then pour onto a plate.
4. Repeat the process with another half tsp of oil and the rest of the dough—top pancakes with walnuts and blueberries.

Nutrition: Calories: 160, Fat: 2g, Carbs: 31g, Protein: 4g

Carrot Muffins

 Prep Time: 10 minutes

 Cooking Time: 20 minutes

 Servings: 8-12

INGREDIENTS

2 eggs
1 tbsp olive oil
1 cup almond milk
2 cups whole wheat flour
¼ tsp baking soda
1 cut carrot
1 tsp cinnamon

DIRECTIONS

1. In a bowl, combine all wet ingredients.
2. In another bowl, combine all dry ingredients. Combine wet and dry ingredients.
3. Pour mixture into 8-12 prepared muffin cups, and fill 2/3 of the cups. Bake for 18-20 minutes at 375 F. Let it cool and serve.

Nutrition: Calories: 34, Fat: 1g, Carbs: 7g, Protein: 0g

Barley Oats Granola with Almond

 Prep Time: 10 minutes

 Cooking Time: 30 minutes

 Servings: 12

INGREDIENTS

1 cup rolled oats
½ cup barley, unco-oked
½ cup almond, chop-ped
¼ cup chia seeds
1/8 tsp salt
3 tbsp olive oil
3 tbsp stevia
1 tsp pure vanilla extract
¼ cup coconut flakes unsweetened

DIRECTIONS

1. Turn the oven to 325 F. Line a baking sheet with parchment paper or a silicone mat.
2. Add the oats, barley, almond, chia seeds, and salt to a medium bowl. Stir to mix. Add the oil, stevia, and vanilla extract. Mix well. Spread on the baking sheet.
3. Bake for 25 minutes on a third rack from the bottom, then sprinkle with coconut flakes and cook for 5 minutes.
4. Take the barley granola out of the oven, let it cool completely (do not touch it), then break it into pieces.

Nutrition: Calories: 137; Fat: 6.7g; Carbs: 16.9g; Protein: 2.9g

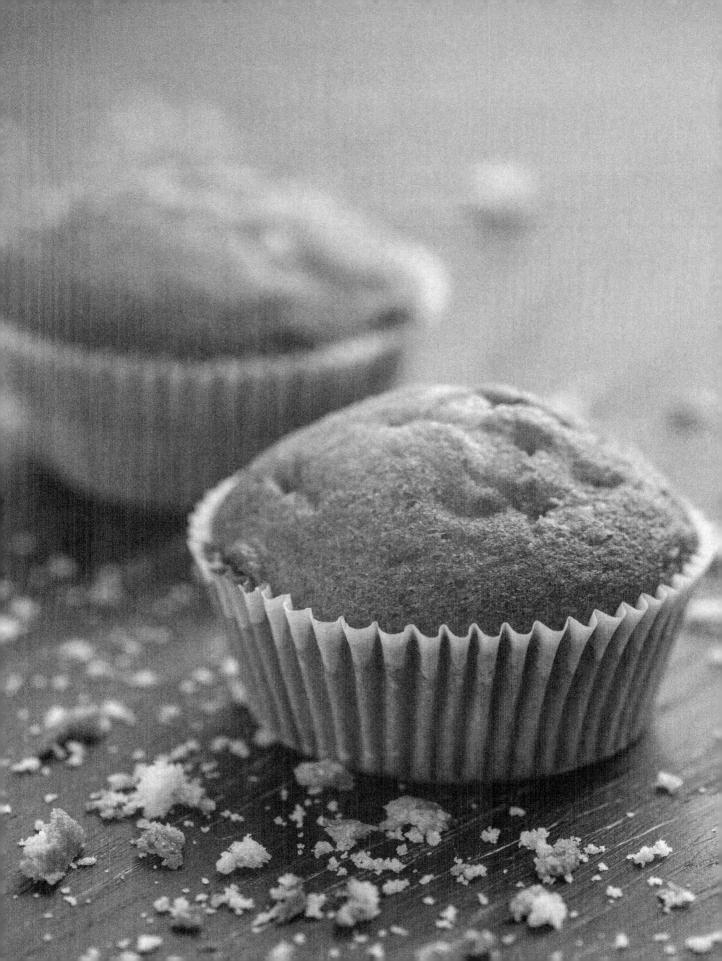

Cabbage Omelet

 Prep Time: 5 minutes

 Cooking Time: 10 minutes

 Servings: 1

INGREDIENTS

2 eggs
¼ tsp salt
¼ tsp black pepper
1 tbsp olive oil
¼ cup nonfat or low-fat cheese
¼ tsp basil
1 cup red onion
1 cup cabbage

DIRECTIONS

1. In your bowl, combine all ingredients and mix well.
2. In a skillet, heat olive oil and pour the egg mixture. Cook for 1-2 minutes per side and serve.

Nutrition: Calories: 20, Fat: 0g, Carbs: 9g, Protein: 4g

Avocado & Pineapple Muffins

 Prep Time: 10 minutes

 Cooking Time: 20 minutes

 Servings: 12

INGREDIENTS

3 eggs, beaten
¼ cup honey
2 tbsp olive oil
2/3 cup ripe avocado, mashed
8 oz canned crushed pineapple
2 cups whole wheat flour
½ tsp baking soda
½ tsp baking powder
½ tsp ground cinnamon
½ tsp salt
¾ cup pecans, toasted and chopped

DIRECTIONS

1. Preheat your oven to 375 F.
2. Mix the eggs, honey, olive oil, and mashed avocado in a bowl. Stir in the crushed pineapple.
3. Combine the all-purpose flour, baking soda, baking powder, ground cinnamon, and salt in another bowl. Add this to the avocado mixture, and fold in the pecans.
4. Pour the mixture into a muffin pan. Bake in the oven within 20 to 30 minutes. Let it cool on a wire rack before serving.

Nutrition: Calories: 103, Fat: 7g, Carbs: 10g, Protein: 1g

Lunch

Chicken Tenders with Pineapple

 Prep Time: 20 minutes   Cooking Time: 10 minutes   Servings: 10

INGREDIENTS

2 pounds of chicken breast strips
1 cup pineapple juice
½ cup honey
1/3 cup light soy sauce

DIRECTIONS

1. Mix the pineapple juice, honey, and soy sauce in a small saucepan over medium heat. Remove from heat just before cooking.
2. Place the chicken fillets in a medium bowl. Cover with the pineapple marinade and store in the refrigerator for at least 30 minutes.
3. Preheat the grill to medium heat. Thread the chicken lengthwise onto wooden skewers.
4. Lightly grease the grill. Grill the chicken fillets for 5 minutes per side or until juices run clear. Serve and enjoy!

Nutrition: Calories: 99; Fat: 1g; Carbs: 20.1g; Protein: 3.7g

---

White Fish Fillets with Sweet Potato Flakes

 Prep Time: 20 minutes   Cooking Time: 10 minutes   Servings: 4

INGREDIENTS

4 white fish fillets
1 free-range egg
1 ½ cups sweet potato, grated
¼ cup olive oil
2 tbsp Dijon mustard
Salt and black pepper to taste

DIRECTIONS

1. Mix the egg, Dijon, salt, and pepper in a shallow bowl. Put the shaved sweet potato in a separate shallow bowl. Heat the olive oil in a heavy-bottomed pan.
2. Meanwhile, dip the fillets in the egg mix, then dredge them in the sweet potato shavings.
3. Dip the fish a second time in your two bowls for a very crisp coating. Fry the fillets for 3-5 minutes per side or until golden and crisp. Serve hot with your salad of choice.

Nutrition: Calories: 199; Fat: 12.5 g; Carbs: 8.7 g; Protein: 16.6 g

Millet Lettuce Wraps

 Prep Time: 10 minutes　　 Cooking Time: 20 minutes　　 Servings: 2

INGREDIENTS

4 leaves lettuce
¼ cup millet
1 tsp nonfat or low-fat butter
½ cup water
¼ red onion, chopped
1 clove of garlic, minced
2 tbsp fresh lime juice
1 tsp chopped cilantro
½ tsp sea salt
1 carrot, chopped

DIRECTIONS

1. In a skillet, toast millet for about 5 minutes or until fragrant and toasted; transfer to a plate and set aside.
2. Add the butter to the skillet and sauté in red onion and garlic for about 3 minutes or until fragrant.
3. Stir in toasted millet, lime juice, cilantro, sea salt, and water; simmer for about 10 minutes or until the liquid is absorbed. Remove from heat.
4. Divide carrots among the lettuce, leave, and top each with the millet mixture. Roll to form wraps and serve.

Nutrition: Calories: 133; Fat: 3 g; Carbs: 19.9 g; Protein: 3.3 g

---

Steamed Chicken with Mushroom & Ginger

 Prep Time: 10 minutes　　 Cooking Time: 10 minutes　　 Servings: 4

INGREDIENTS

4 chicken breast fillets
2 tsp extra-virgin olive oil
1 1/2 tbsp balsamic vinegar
1 (3-inch) ginger, cut into matchsticks
1 bunch broccoli
1 bunch of carrots, diced
6 small dried shiitake mushrooms, chopped
Spring onion, sliced, as you like
Fresh coriander leaves, as you like

DIRECTIONS

1. In a bowl, mix sliced chicken with salt, vinegar, and pepper; let marinate for at least 10 minutes.
2. Move the chicken to your baking dish and top with mushrooms and ginger; bake for about 15 minutes in a preheated oven at 350 F.
3. Top with chopped broccoli and carrots and return to the oven. Cook within 3 minutes or until chicken is tender.
4. Divide the chicken, broccoli, and carrots on serving plates and drizzle each with olive oil, and top with coriander and red onions. Serve!

Nutrition: Calories: 242; Fat: 5g; Carbs: 10g; Protein: 37 g

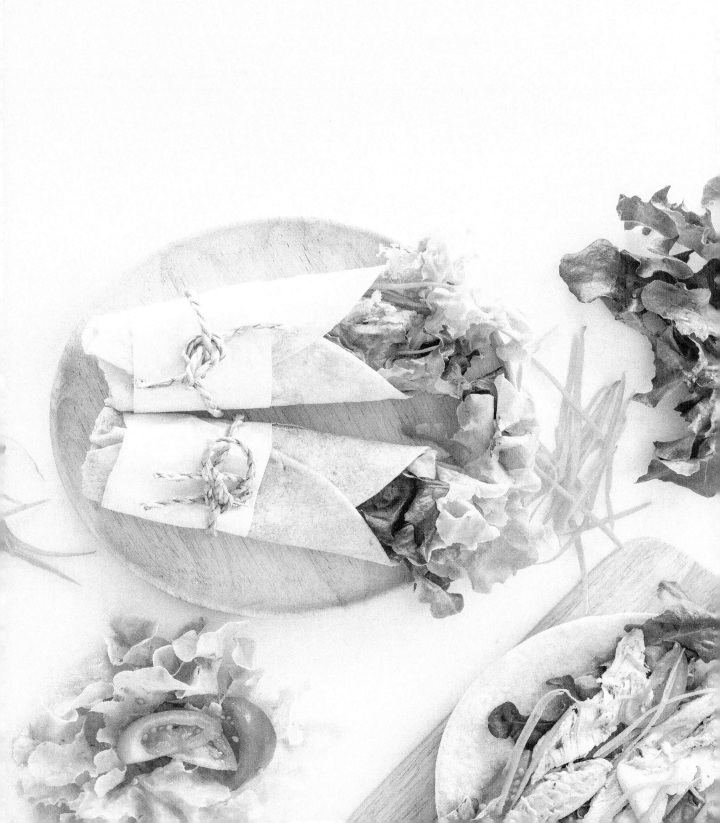

Grilled Turkey Teriyaki

 Prep Time: 15 minutes Cooking Time: 10-15 minutes Servings: 4

INGREDIENTS

4 (6 ounces) turkey breast
2 tbsp coconut aminos
1 tbsp apple cider vinegar
1 tbsp minced fresh ginger root
1 large clove of garlic, minced
1 tbsp olive oil

DIRECTIONS

1. Mix the coconut aminos, apple cider vinegar, ginger, and garlic in a shallow bowl.
2. Put the turkey breast in the marinade and turn it over to coat it. Cover the plate and refrigerate for at least 30 to 45 minutes.
3. Preheat the grill. Remove the breast out of the marinade. Discard any remaining liquid. Coat both sides of your meat with oil.
4. Cook the turkey breast on the preheated grill for 10 to 15 minutes per side until cooked through. Serve with herbs, rice, or veggies of your choice.

Nutrition: Calories: 217; Fat: 6.3g; Carbs: 9.1g; Protein: 29.1g

---

Glazed Tempeh

 Prep Time: 5 minutes Cooking Time: 15 minutes Servings: 8

INGREDIENTS

2 pounds tempeh, trimmed
2 tbsp olive oil
½ cup apple cider vinegar
4 tbsp pure maple syrup
2 tbsp Dijon mustard

DIRECTIONS

1. Cut the tempeh into 1-inch slices. Using your medium-sized pan, heat the olive oil until it begins to melt.
2. In the meantime, preheat the oven to 375 F and spray a baking sheet with non-stick cooking spray.
3. Fry the tempeh for a minute on each side and place them on a baking sheet.
4. Whisk the vinegar, maple syrup, and Dijon mustard in a small bowl. Generously brush the tempeh with the glaze—Bake for 10 minutes and serve.

Nutrition: Calories: 280; Fat: 5.8g; Carbs: 17.7g; Protein: 21.2g

Cod Parcels with Mushrooms and Spinach

 Prep Time: 15 minutes   Cooking Time: 15 minutes   Servings: 4

INGREDIENTS

4 (4-ounce) cod fillets
4 cups of baby spinach
2 cups sliced shiitake mushrooms
½ tsp Old Bay seasoning
½ tsp salt
¼ tsp freshly ground black pepper
¼ cup chopped scallions, green and white parts
2 tbsp extra-virgin olive oil

DIRECTIONS

1. Preheat the oven to 425 F.
2. Tear 4 (12-inch) square pieces of aluminum foil. Place 1 cup of spinach and ½ cup of mushrooms into each piece of foil.
3. Place 1 piece of cod on top—season with the Old Bay, salt, and pepper.
4. Sprinkle with the scallions, then drizzle with the oil. Fold up the packets to seal and enclose the cod.
5. Place the packets on a baking sheet. Transfer your baking sheet to the oven, and bake for 15 minutes. Remove from the oven. Carefully unfold the packets and serve.

Nutrition: Calories: 155; Fat: 7g; Carbs: 3g; Protein: 19g

Sautéed Turkey with Cabbage

 Prep Time: 10 minutes   Cooking Time: 20 minutes   Servings: 4

INGREDIENTS

2 turkey breasts, skinless, boneless, and sliced
1 head of cabbage, shredded
2 carrots, shredded
3 tomatoes, pureed
1 cup chicken stock
2 tbsp olive oil
sea salt & freshly ground black pepper, as needed

DIRECTIONS

1. Heat the olive oil in a skillet over medium heat. Cook the turkey slices until golden brown on each side.
2. When you are almost done, add the shredded cabbage and carrots to the pan and cook, stirring, for 4-5 minutes.
3. Add the tomatoes and chicken broth, and season to taste. Stir the content well, then bring it to a boil.
4. Adjust the heat to low and simmer for 10-12 minutes to ensure the turkey is cooked through. Remove from the heat and serve hot.

Nutrition: Calories: 172; Fat: 8.3g; Carbs: 20.9g; Protein: 7.9g

Chicken Souvlaki Kebabs

 Prep Time: 10 minutes   Cooking Time: 15 minutes   Servings: 4

INGREDIENTS

1-pound boneless, skinless chicken breasts, cut into 1-inch dice
Juice of 1 lemon
2 tbsp extra-virgin olive oil
5 garlic cloves, minced
1 tsp dried rosemary
1 tsp dried oregano
½ tsp salt
¼ tsp freshly ground black pepper

DIRECTIONS

1. Combine the chicken, lemon juice, oil, garlic, rosemary, oregano, salt, and pepper in your medium bowl. Let rest for 30 minutes.
2. Thread the chicken pieces onto 8 skewers. Warm a grill on medium-high heat, or preheat a grill pan over medium-high heat.
3. Put the skewers on the grill, and cook for 5 to 7 minutes. Flip, cook for 5 to 8 minutes, or until cooked through and browned. Remove from the heat.

Nutrition: Calories: 205; Fat: 10g; Carbs: 2g; Protein: 26g

Baked Lemon Salmon with Zucchini

 Prep Time: 10 minutes   Cooking Time: 20 minutes   Servings: 1

INGREDIENTS

1 zucchini
1 onion
1 scallion
1 salmon fillet
1 tsp lemon zest
1 tsp olive oil
Lemon slices, as you like

DIRECTIONS

1. Preheat the oven to 375 F.
2. Add zucchini and onion, and sprinkle vegetables with salt and lemon zest in a baking dish. Lay salmon fillet and season with salt, lemon zest, and olive oil.
3. Bake at 375 F for 15-18 minutes, remove and serve with lemon slices.

Nutrition: Calories: 160, Carbs: 1g, Fat: 7g, Protein: 22g

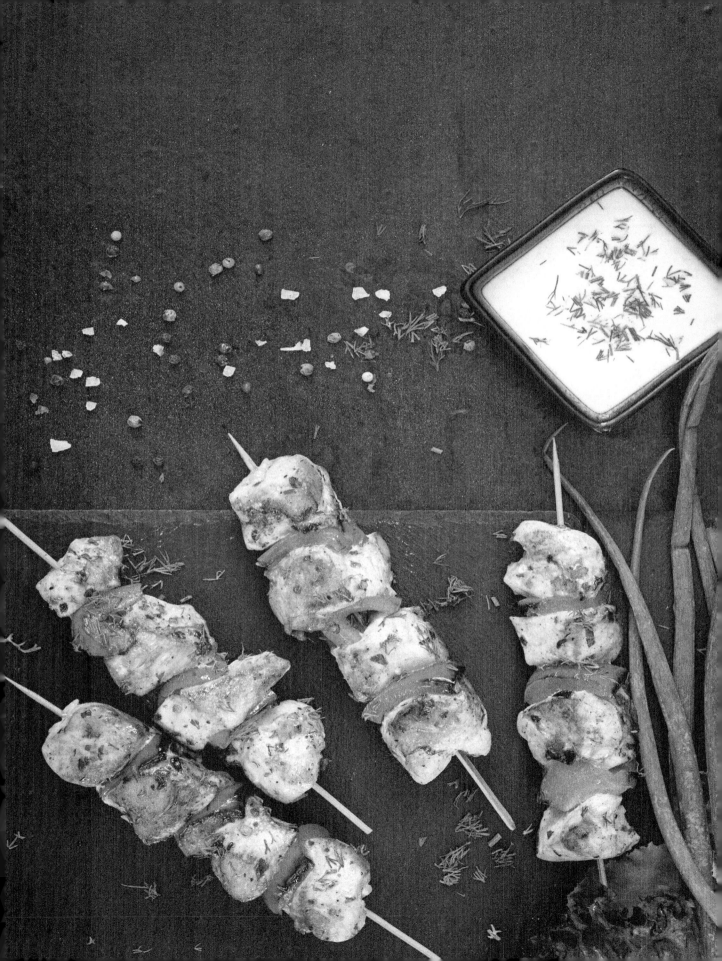

Chicken And Rice

 Prep Time: 10 minutes   Cooking Time: 20 minutes   Servings: 4

INGREDIENTS

2 lb. chicken thighs
1 cup rice
15 oz salsa
3 tsp salt
3 tbs olive oil
1 ½ cup low-sodium
chicken broth

DIRECTIONS

1. Cut the chicken and toss with the salt. Cook in hot oil until browned.
2. Add the rice and mix well, cooking 1 more minute to toast the rice. Add the broth and salsa and stir.
3. Let it simmer, cover and cook within 20 minutes, Serve immediately!

Nutrition: Calories: 160, Carbs: 27g, Fat: 3g, Protein: 7g

Turkey Salad

 Prep Time: 5 minutes   Cooking Time: 5 minutes   Servings: 2

INGREDIENTS

2 tbsp lemon juice
2 tbsp roasted garlic
2 tbsp olive oil
1 tbsp honey
2 cups cooked turkey breast
1 cup berries
1 cup green onions
Nonfat or low-fat
Salad dressing of your choice, as you like

DIRECTIONS

1. In a bowl, combine all ingredients and mix well.
2. Serve with dressing.

Nutrition: Calories: 160, Carbs: 2g, Fat: 7g, Protein: 7g

Chickpea Veggie Sauté

 Prep Time: 5 minutes   Cooking Time: 15 minutes   Servings: 4

INGREDIENTS

2 tbsp extra-virgin olive oil
3 garlic cloves, minced
1 (15- oz) can of low-so-dium chickpeas, drained and rinsed
1 (15-oz) can of low-so-dium diced tomatoes
½ tsp salt
¼ tsp freshly ground black pepper
4 cups of baby spinach

DIRECTIONS

1. In your large skillet, heat the oil over medium heat. Add the garlic, and cook for 30 seconds, or until fragrant.
2. Add the chickpeas and tomatoes with their juices, salt, and pepper. Bring to a simmer. Cook, stirring regularly, within 10 minutes or until the flavors meld.
3. Add the spinach, and stir within 1 to 2 minutes, or until wilted. Remove from the heat.

Nutrition: Calories: 168; Fat: 9g; Carbs: 18g; Protein: 6g

Ginger Glazed Tuna

 Prep Time: 5 minutes   Cooking Time: 15 minutes   Servings: 2

INGREDIENTS

1 ½ tbsp maple syrup
1 ½ tbsp coconut aminos
1 ½ tbsp apple cider vinegar
½ tsp grated fresh ginger root
½ tsp garlic powder
1 tsp olive oil
2 (6 ounces) tuna fillets
salt and pepper to taste
½ tbsp avocado oil

DIRECTIONS

1. Mix the maple syrup, coconut aminos, apple cider vinegar, ginger, garlic powder, and olive oil in a small glass bowl.
2. Place the fillets on a plate and sprinkle salt and pepper—cover to marinate and refrigerate for 20 minutes.
3. Heath the oil in a skillet over medium heat. Remove the fish from the plate and keep the marinade. Bake the fish on a pan for 4 to 6 minutes per side, turning it just once, until tender.
4. Place the steaks on a platter. Keep them warm. Heat the remaining marinade into the skillet over medium heat until the mixture is evenly reduced to a glaze.
5. Pour it over the fillets and serve immediately. If desired, serve with some brown rice.

Nutrition: Calories: 88; Fat: 2.8g; Carbs: 7.6g; Protein: 7.7g

Buddha Bowl

 Prep Time: 10 minutes   Cooking Time: 10 minutes   Servings: 1

INGREDIENTS

1 zucchini
¼ tsp oregano
Salt, as needed
1 cup cooked quinoa
1 cup spinach
1 cup mixed greens
½ cup red pepper
¼ cup cucumber
¼ cup tomatoes
Parsley, as you like
Tahini dressing, as you like

DIRECTIONS

1. Heat olive oil olive and sauté zucchini in a skillet until soft; sprinkle oregano over zucchini.
2. Add the rest of the fixings to a bowl and toss to combine. Add fried zucchini and mix well.
3. Pour over tahini dressing, mix well and serve.

Nutrition: Calories: 135, Carbs: 19g, Fat: 4g, Protein: 4g

Cauliflower Shawarma with Tahini

 Prep Time: 5 minutes   Cooking Time: 30 minutes   Servings: 4

INGREDIENTS

1 head cauliflower, cut into florets
2 tbsp extra-virgin olive oil
½ tsp ground coriander
1 tsp ground cumin
Salt & freshly ground black pepper, as needed
½ cup Tahini Dressing

DIRECTIONS

1. Warm the oven to 400 F. Line a baking sheet with parchment paper.
2. Toss together the cauliflower, oil, coriander, and cumin in a large bowl. Season lightly with salt and pepper.
3. Spread your cauliflower out in a single layer on the prepared baking sheet.
4. Transfer your baking sheet to the oven, and bake for 25 to 30 minutes, or until the cauliflower is tender. Remove from the oven. Drizzle with the dressing.

Nutrition: Calories: 50, Carbs: 11g, Fat: 5g, Protein: 4g

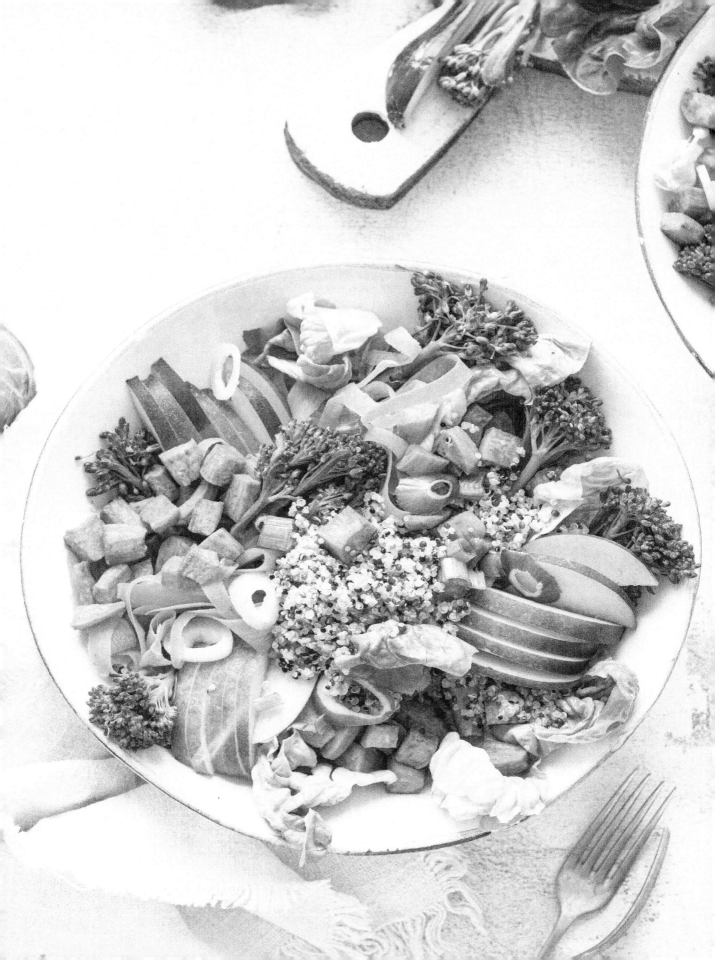

Kale and Cottage Pasta

 Prep Time: 5 minutes   Cooking Time: 15 minutes   Servings: 4

INGREDIENTS

1 oz gluten-free elbow macaroni or any type
1 tsp olive oil
¼ cup onion, finely chopped
1 garlic clove, minced
5 cups fresh kale, roughly chopped
½ oz fresh parsley, chopped
½ cup nonfat or low-fat cottage cheese
1/8 cup coconut milk

DIRECTIONS

1. Cook pasta according to package instructions.
2. Dissolve the olive oil in a saucepan over medium heat. Add onion and garlic and sauté until onions are tender and fragrant, within 5 minutes.
3. Add parsley and the kale to the pan and stir until tender. Add the cottage cheese and coconut milk to the saucepan and stir well.
4. Drain the pasta and keep about ¼ cup of the cooking water. Mix cooked pasta and cottage mixture in a large bowl. Serve immediately with freshly ground black pepper.

Nutrition: Calories: 125; Fat: 3.7g; Carbs: 16.4g; Protein: 7.7g

---

Chicken and Cauliflower Rice Bowls

 Prep Time: 10 minutes   Cooking Time: 20 minutes   Servings: 4

INGREDIENTS

½ tsp Italian seasoning
½ tsp salt
¼ cup freshly ground black pepper
2 tbsp extra-virgin olive oil, divided
4 cups cauliflower rice
1 (15-oz) can of artichoke hearts, drained
¼ cup chopped Kalamata olives

DIRECTIONS

1. Season your chicken with Italian seasoning, salt, plus pepper.
2. In your large skillet, heat 1 tablespoon of oil over medium-high heat. Add the chicken, and cook within 3 to 5 minutes, or until browned.
3. Flip your chicken, and cook on the other side for 3 to 5 minutes, or until cooked through. Transfer to a cutting board. Thinly slice the chicken across the grain.
4. Heat the rest of your oil in your same skillet over medium-high heat.
5. Add the cauliflower rice, and cook for 5 to 8 minutes, or until tender.
6. Add the artichoke hearts and olives. Mix well to heat through. Remove from the heat. Serve the cauliflower and vegetables topped with the chicken.

Nutrition: Calories: 270; Fat: 11g; Carbs: 14g; Protein: 30g

Italian Fish Fillet

 Prep Time: 10 minutes   Cooking Time: 0 minutes   Servings: 4

INGREDIENTS

4 tilapia fillets
Pepper to taste
14 oz. canned diced to-matoes with herbs
1 green pepper, sliced thinly
1 onion, sliced thinly
¼ cup nonfat or low-fat Parmesan cheese, shred-ded

DIRECTIONS

1. Preheat your oven to 350 F.
2. Arrange the tilapia fillets in a baking pan and season with pepper. Top with the tomatoes, green pepper, and onion.
3. Cover the baking pan with foil. Bake in the oven for 30 minutes. Sprinkle the parmesan cheese on top. Bake within 10 minutes or until the fish is flaky, and serve!

Nutrition: Calories: 130, Carbs: 0g, Fat: 7g, Protein: 16g

Smashed Chickpea Salad Sandwich

 Prep Time: 10 minutes   Cooking Time: 0 minutes   Servings: 4

INGREDIENTS

1 (15-oz) can of chi-ckpeas, low-sodium, drained and rinsed
¼ cup finely chopped red onion
¼ cup plain nonfat or low-fat Greek yogurt, unsweetened
1½ tsp whole-grain mustard
Salt & freshly ground black pepper, as nee-ded
4 whole-grain bread slices

DIRECTIONS

1. Using a fork, mash the chickpeas coarsely in your bowl, leaving some whole for texture.
2. Add the onion, yogurt, and mustard—season with salt and pepper.
3. Divide the salad between 2 pieces of bread. Top with the remaining slices of bread.

Nutrition: Calories: 162; Fat: 3g; Carbs: 26g; Protein: 8g

Chicken Fajita Bowl

 Prep Time: 10 minutes   Cooking Time: 10 minutes   Servings: 4

INGREDIENTS

1 ½ pounds chicken breasts cut into bite size pieces
1 ½ tsp oregano
½ tsp garlic, minced
½ tsp onion powder
1 ½ tsp salt
¾ tsp black pepper
1 ½ tsp cumin
½ tsp basil
1 large onion diced
1 yellow or orange bell pepper diced
1 ½ tbsp olive oil

DIRECTIONS

1. Mix oregano, onion powder, garlic, salt, black pepper, cumin, and basil in a small bowl until well blended.
2. Pour a tbsp of olive oil into your saucepan and add the chicken and half of the spice mixer.
3. Stir often until your meat is cooked through within 5-7 minutes and transfer to your plate.
4. Add the rest of the oil, onion, and peppers to the pan. Spread the rest of the spice mixer on top and cook, for about 8 to 10 minutes, until tender.
5. Serve the chicken, peppers, and onions over romaine lettuce or cauliflower rice and garnish with avocado if desired.

Nutrition: Calories: 332; Fat: 9.3g; Carbs: 9.8g; Protein: 50.9g

---

Tuna Melt Stuffed Tomatoes

 Prep Time: 5 minutes   Cooking Time: 5 minutes   Servings: 2

INGREDIENTS

6 oz tuna
3 tbsp onion
¼ tsp salt
¼ tsp black pepper
1 avocado
3 tbsp nonfat or low-fat Greek yogurt
3 oz nonfat or low-fat cheese
2 tomatoes

DIRECTIONS

1. Mix onion, tuna, diced avocado, Greek yogurt, salt, and pepper.
2. Place tomato slices on a baking sheet on a wire rack.
3. To each slice with tuna mixture, then top with cheese. Broil until cheese is melted, and serve!

Nutrition: Calories: 144, Carbs: 15g, Fat: 1g, Protein: 19g

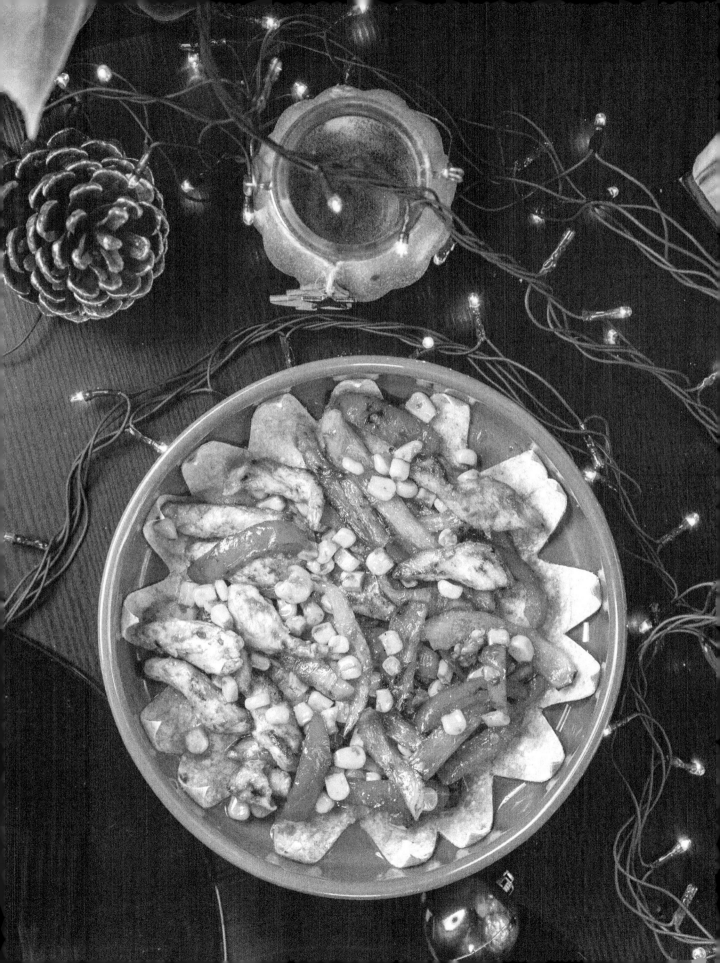

Watercress Sandwich

 Prep Time: 10 minutes   Cooking Time: 20 minutes   Servings: 4

INGREDIENTS

8 free-range eggs, hardboiled, peeled & cut in half
4 green onions, sliced
4 tbsp nonfat or low-fat Greek yogurt, unsweetened
¾ cup watercress stems removed and cleaned
1 tbsp Dijon mustard
Salt and black pepper to taste
8 slice wholemeal bread

DIRECTIONS

1. Separate the egg yolks from the whites and chop all the whites. Mash two yolks in a small bowl and mix the Greek yogurt and Dijon mustard.
2. Mix the chopped egg whites with the onions and season with salt and pepper. Roughly chop the remaining yolks and add to the egg white mix. Mix in the yogurt mix and mix well.
3. Set out four slices of bread and top with watercress leaves and egg salad. Cover with the remaining slices. Slice diagonally and serve!

Nutrition: Calories: 158; Fat: 10.1 g; Carbs: 13.3 g; Protein: 6.2 g

---

Chicken and Brussels Sprouts Skillet

 Prep Time: 5 minutes   Cooking Time: 25 minutes   Servings: 4

INGREDIENTS

4 bone-in chicken thighs, skin removed
1 pound Brussels sprouts, trimmed and halved
½ tsp salt, divided
¼ tsp freshly ground black pepper
2 tbsp extra-virgin olive oil
1 onion, cut into half-moons
1 cup low-sodium vegetable broth
Juice of 1 lemon

DIRECTIONS

1. Preheat the oven to 350 F.
2. Season the chicken with ½ teaspoon of salt and pepper.
3. In your large oven-safe skillet, heat the oil over medium-high heat. Place the chicken in your skillet so that the side that had skin faces the bottom, and sear within 3 to 5 minutes, or until browned, then flip.
4. Scatter the onion plus Brussels sprouts around the chicken. Add the stock, and let it simmer. Turn off the heat.
5. Transfer your skillet to the oven, then bake within 20 minutes, or until cooked through. Remove from the oven.
6. Sprinkle the lemon juice over the top of the chicken and Brussels sprouts.

Nutrition: Calories: 275; Fat: 12g; Carbs: 17g; Protein: 27g

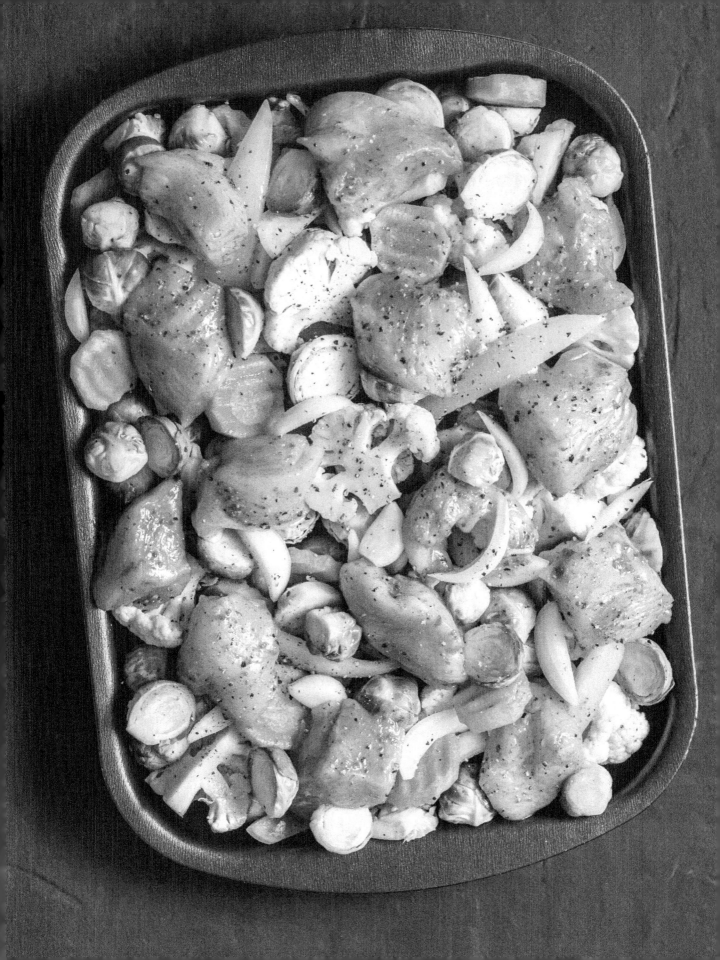

Salmon Burgers

 Prep Time: 10 minutes   Cooking Time: 10 minutes   Servings: 12

INGREDIENTS

1 lb. salmon, cut into cubes
3 eggs
2 tbsp whole wheat flour
½ cup sesame seeds
4 tbsp olive oil
2 tbsp vinegar
2 garlic cloves
2 tsp ginger
½ cup scallions

DIRECTIONS

1. Mix the eggs, vinegar, scallions, 2 tbsp oil, ginger, sesame seeds, and ginger. Add the salmon, then stir in the flour. Form the mixture into patties.
2. Heat the rest of the oil in a frying pan. Cook the patties within 5 minutes on each side. Serve immediately.

Nutrition: Calories: 130, Carbs: 0g, Fat: 6g, Protein: 21g

Artichoke Heart and Chickpea–Stuffed Portabellas

 Prep Time: 10 minutes   Cooking Time: 30 minutes   Servings: 4

INGREDIENTS

4 large portabella mushrooms, stemmed
1 tbsp extra-virgin olive oil
1 (15-oz) can of low-sodium chickpeas, drained and rinsed
1 cup cooked brown rice
½ red bell pepper, cored and finely chopped
½ cup chopped artichoke hearts
Salt & freshly ground black pepper, as needed

DIRECTIONS

1. Preheat the oven to 350 F.
2. Place the mushrooms, gill-side down, on a large baking sheet. Drizzle with the oil.
3. Transfer your baking sheet to the oven, and bake for 10 minutes. Flip the mushrooms, and bake for 10 minutes, or until tender. Remove, leaving the oven on.
4. Combine the chickpeas, rice, bell pepper, and artichoke hearts in your large bowl. Season it with salt and pepper.
5. Divide the mixture among the mushrooms. Return your baking sheet to the oven, then bake for 10 more minutes, or until the filling is heated. Remove from the oven and serve.

Nutrition: Calories: 194; Fat: 6g; Carbs: 29g; Protein: 8g

Chicken Pizza

 Prep Time: 10 minutes   Cooking Time: 20 minutes   Servings: 4

INGREDIENTS

1 ½ tbsp basil
1 cup low-sodium pizza sauce
6 chicken strips
1 10-ounces garlic bread
1 ½ cup nonfat or low-fat cheese

DIRECTIONS

1. Warm the oven to 400 F. Place the garlic bread on a baking sheet.
2. Bake for 10 minutes, then spread the sauce over. Cut the chicken strips and arrange them over.
3. Sprinkle with cheese and basil. Bake until the cheese melts, and serve.

Nutrition: Calories: 190, Carbs: 29g, Fat: 6g, Protein: 11g

Shrimp with Mushrooms

 Prep Time: 10 minutes   Cooking Time: 5 minutes   Servings: 4

INGREDIENTS

2 tsp olive oil
4 cloves garlic, minced
1 lb. shrimp, peeled and deveined
1 cup green onions, chopped
3 cups fresh mushrooms, sliced
¼ cup low-sodium chicken broth
Hot cooked rice, as needed
Lemon wedges, as you like

DIRECTIONS

1. Pour the oil into your pan over medium heat. Cook the garlic for 1 minute, stirring often.
2. Stir in the shrimp, green onions, and mushrooms. Cook while stirring for 1 minute.
3. Pour in the chicken broth—Cook for 2 minutes. Serve with the cooked rice, then garnish with the lemon wedges.

Nutrition: Calories: 245, Carbs: 44g, Fat: 2g, Protein: 12g

Poached Fish in Tomato-Caper Sauce

 Prep Time:5 minutes   Cooking Time: 30 minutes   Servings: 4

INGREDIENTS

1 pound cod or halibut fillets
1 (28-oz) can of low-sodium diced tomatoes
¼ cup capers, drained, rinsed, and finely chopped
3 garlic cloves, minced
½ tsp salt
¼ tsp freshly ground black pepper

DIRECTIONS

1. Combine the tomatoes with their juices, capers, garlic, salt, and pepper in a large saucepan.
2. Bring to a simmer over medium heat. Cook, occasionally stirring, within 15 minutes or until thickened.
3. Using a spatula, slide the fillets into the saucepan, and cook for 10 to 15 minutes until they flake easily with a fork. Remove from the heat.

Nutrition: Calories: 130; Fat: 1g; Carbs: 8g; Protein: 22g

Quinoa Pilaf with Apricots and Pistachios

 Prep Time: 15 minutes   Cooking Time: 15 minutes   Servings: 4

INGREDIENTS

2 shallots, peeled and diced small
1 red bell pepper, medium, seeded, and diced small
¼ cup pistachios, toasted
4 cups cooked quinoa, made with 4 cups low-sodium vegetable broth
¾ cup dried unsulfured apricots, chopped
3 tbsps. chopped mint
Zest and juice of 1 orange
Salt, as needed

DIRECTIONS

1. Put shallots and red pepper in a saucepan and sauté for 10 minutes over medium heat.
2. Pour water 1 tbsp at a time to keep the vegetables from sticking to the pan.
3. Add the quinoa, mint, orange zest and juice, plus apricots and cook about 5 minutes until heated through.
4. Season with salt and garnish with the pistachios.

Nutrition: Calories: 348, Fat: 7.4g, Carbs: 62.11g, Protein: 11.14g

Dinner

Garlic Turkey Breasts with Lemon

 Prep Time: 10 minutes   Cooking Time: 25 minutes   Servings: 2

INGREDIENTS

1 tsp garlic powder
2 skinless turkey breast halves
salt and ground black pepper to taste
½ cup low-sodium chicken broth
½ tbsp lemon juice
1 tbsp chopped cilantro

DIRECTIONS

1. Place the nonstick skillet over low heat.
2. Season the breast with garlic powder, salt, and pepper and place it on a skillet. Cook over medium heat, 10 to 12 minutes, until golden brown on both sides.
3. Pour in the chicken broth and let it boil, lower to medium-low heat, add the lemon juice, cover, and cook within 10 to 15 minutes, or until the breast is no longer pink in the center.
4. Place the breast on the serving platter and keep the liquid in the pan. Simmer the liquid for about 3 minutes until slightly reduced. Pour liquid over the breast. Garnish with fresh cilantro before serving.

Nutrition: Calories: 158; Fat: 4.7g; Carbs: 1.4g; Protein: 26.5g

---

Red Lentil Soup with Tomato Sauce

 Prep Time: 10 minutes   Cooking Time: 20 minutes   Servings: 4

INGREDIENTS

2 tsp olive oil
2 (15-oz) cans of low-salt red or brown lentils, drained
1 (15-oz) can of low-salt tomato sauce
1 cup onion, chopped
1 cup celery, chopped
2 cups carrots, chopped
¼ tsp. pepper, freshly ground
¼ cup cilantro, chopped fresh
4 cups water

DIRECTIONS

1. Heat oil in your large pot over medium-high heat. Put in onion, carrot, and celery. Cook for about 6 minutes until vegetables begin to soften.
2. Add tomato sauce, pepper, lentils, and water. After the low boil, reduce heat and simmer for 15 minutes, or until vegetables are tender.
3. Ladle into bowls and top with cilantro. Serve.

Nutrition: Calories: 150, Fat: 1g, Carbs: 28g, Protein: 8g

Baked Flounder with Tomatoes and Basil

 Prep Time: 10 minutes   Cooking Time: 20 minutes   Servings: 4

INGREDIENTS

4 (5- to 6-oz) flounder fillets
1 pound of cherry tomatoes
4 garlic cloves, sliced
2 tbsp extra-virgin olive oil
2 tbsp lemon juice
2 tbsp basil, cut into ribbons
½ tsp kosher salt
¼ tsp freshly ground black pepper

DIRECTIONS

1. Preheat the oven to 425 F.
2. Combine the tomatoes, garlic, olive oil, lemon juice, basil, salt, and black pepper in a baking dish and mix well. Bake for 5 minutes.
3. Remove your baking dish and arrange the flounder on the tomato mixture.
4. Bake until the fish is opaque and flakes, about 10 to 15 minutes, depending on thickness.

Nutrition: Calories: 215, Fat: 9g, Carbs: 6g, Protein: 28g

Baked Mustard-Lime Chicken

 Prep Time: 10 minutes   Cooking Time: 20 minutes   Servings: 4

INGREDIENTS

¼ cup freshly squeezed lime juice
¼ cup chopped fresh cilantro
2 garlic cloves, minced
2 tbsp Dijon mustard
½ tbsp olive oil
1/8 tsp salt
¼ tsp freshly ground black pepper
2 (4-oz) skinless, boneless chicken breasts

DIRECTIONS

1. Preheat the oven to 350 F.
2. Add the lime juice, cilantro, garlic, mustard, olive oil, salt, and pepper to a food processor and pulse until the fixings are well combined.
3. Place the chicken breasts in a 7-by-11-inch glass oven-proof baking dish. Pour the marinade over the chicken, cover, and refrigerate for at least 15 minutes or 6 hours.
4. Bake, uncovered, within 18 to 20 minutes, or until an instant-read thermometer registers 165°F. Serve immediately.

Nutrition: Calories: 189; Fats: 5g; Carbs: 4g; Protein: 27g

Buckwheat with Mushrooms & Green Onions

 Prep Time: 20 minutes   Cooking Time: 35 minutes   Servings: 6

INGREDIENTS

1 cup uncooked buckwheat
2 cup water
2 cups mushrooms
1 red onion, chopped
1 cup chopped green onions
3 tbsp olive oil
A pinch of salt and pepper

DIRECTIONS

1. Mix buckwheat, salt, and water in a pan, bring to a boil, and cook for 25 minutes or until liquid is absorbed.
2. Put the olive oil in a pan and fry in red onion until tender; stir in mushrooms and cook within 5 minutes or until golden brown.
3. Stir in cooked buckwheat and remove from heat. Serve topped with freshly chopped green onions.

Nutrition: Calories: 166; Fat: 6.8 g; Carbs: 20.1 g; Protein: 5.1 g

---

Seafood Fettuccine

 Prep Time: 15 minutes   Cooking Time: 20 minutes   Servings: 4

INGREDIENTS

1 tbsp olive oil
½ pound cooked bay shrimp
½ pound cooked crab
10 ounces dry fettuccine noodles
3 tbsp minced garlic
2 medium tomatoes, sliced into bite-sized pieces
1 green bell pepper, sliced into bite-sized pieces
2 tbsp chopped fresh basil
2 tbsp chopped fresh oregano

DIRECTIONS

1. Boil the fettuccine per package directions. Meanwhile, combine the garlic plus oil in a large nonstick skillet and heat gently over medium heat. Add the tomatoes and peppers to the skillet.
2. Stir in the basil and oregano, add the shrimp and crab, and cook until the seafood is heated. Drain your pasta and stir it into your skillet, coating thoroughly. Serve and enjoy!

Nutrition: Calories: 569, Fat: 12.17g, Carbs: 99.5g, Protein: 28.26g

Pasta and Fagioli

 Prep Time: 10 minutes   Cooking Time: 15 minutes   Servings: 4

INGREDIENTS

8 oz rotini pasta
2 tbsp extra-virgin olive oil
1 bunch kale, stemmed and chopped
1 (15-oz) can of low-sodium diced tomatoes, drained
1 (15- oz) can of low-sodium white beans, drained and rinsed
1 tsp dried oregano
Salt & freshly ground black pepper

DIRECTIONS

1. Fill a large saucepan with water. Bring to a boil.
2. Cook the pasta as stated in the package directions until al dente. Remove from the heat. Reserve about ½ cup of the cooking water, then drain.
3. In your large skillet, heat the oil over medium-high heat. Add the kale, and sauté for 4 to 6 minutes, or until wilted.
4. Add the tomatoes and beans. Cook within 3 to 5 minutes, or until heated through and the tomatoes release some of their water. Season with the oregano, salt, and pepper.
5. Stir the pasta into your skillet along with ¼ cup of the cooking water. Continue cooking, stirring for 1 more minute, or until heated through. Remove and serve!

Nutrition: Calories: 435; Fat: 9g; Carbs: 73g; Protein: 18g

Orange Maple Glazed Salmon

 Prep Time: 10 minutes   Cooking Time: 15 minutes   Servings: 4

INGREDIENTS

4 (4- to 6-oz) salmon fillets, pin bones removed
¼ cup pure maple syrup
juice of 2 oranges
zest of 1 orange
2 tbsp low-sodium soy sauce
1 tsp garlic powder

DIRECTIONS

1. Preheat the oven to 400 F.
2. Add the maple syrup, orange juice and zest, soy sauce, and garlic powder into a small, shallow dish, and whisk them together well.
3. Flesh-side down to put the salmon pieces into the dish. Allow it to marinate for 10 minutes.
4. Then skin-side up, transfer the salmon to a rimmed baking sheet and bake until the flesh is opaque about 15 minutes.

Nutrition: Calories: 297, Fat: 11, Carbs: 18g, Protein: 34g

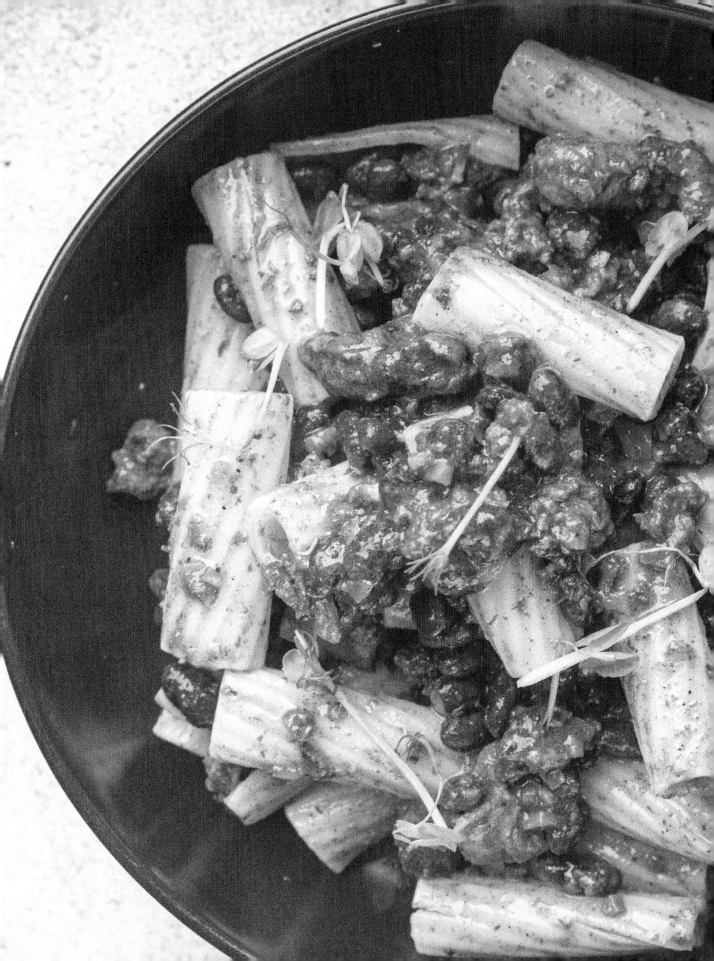

Cheesy Tortilla Casserole

 Prep Time: 15 minutes   Cooking Time: 20 minutes   Servings: 2

INGREDIENTS

1 cup organic salsa
2 tbsp olive oil
½ canned of refried beans
1 sweet onion, diced
½ cup nonfat or low-fat ricotta cheese
3 gluten-free tortillas

DIRECTIONS

1. Warm your oven to 375 F. Coat a nonstick pan with olive oil.
2. Cook the onions in a pan over medium heat until soft; add the refried beans and cook for 5 minutes.
3. Spread a tortilla at the base of the prepared pan and spread one-third of the bean mixture, followed by the salsa and the cheese. Repeat with the remaining tortillas, beans, salsa, and cheese.
4. Bake within 15 minutes or until the cheese melts beautifully. Serve and enjoy!

Nutrition: Calories: 302; Fat: 13.4 g; Carbs: 22.1 g; Protein: 20.1 g

---

Chicken with Broccoli Stir-Fry

 Prep Time: 10 minutes   Cooking Time: 15 minutes   Servings: 4

INGREDIENTS

2 boneless, skinless chicken breasts, cubed
2 tbsp olive oil, divided
3 small carrots, thinly sliced
15 oz frozen chopped broccoli florets, thawed
8 oz sliced water chestnuts, drained and thoroughly rinsed
2 garlic cloves, minced
2 tsp ground ginger
3 tbsp balsamic vinegar, divided

DIRECTIONS

1. In a large sauté pan, add ½ tablespoon olive oil and heat over medium heat. Place the cubed chicken and fried about 5 to 7 minutes until lightly browned and cooked through.
2. Transfer chicken from the pan to your bowl with a lid and set aside.
3. Pour the olive oil, garlic, and carrots into the pan and heat over medium heat until the carrots soften, within 3 to 4 minutes.
4. Place the thawed broccoli florets, water chestnuts, and balsamic vinegar into it and cook another for 3 to 4 minutes.
5. Mix the cooked chicken with 2 tbsp balsamic vinegar and 2 tsp ground ginger and stir until well coated. Serve over brown rice if you want, and enjoy.

Nutrition: Calories: 189, Fat: 9g, Carbs: 12g, Protein: 14g

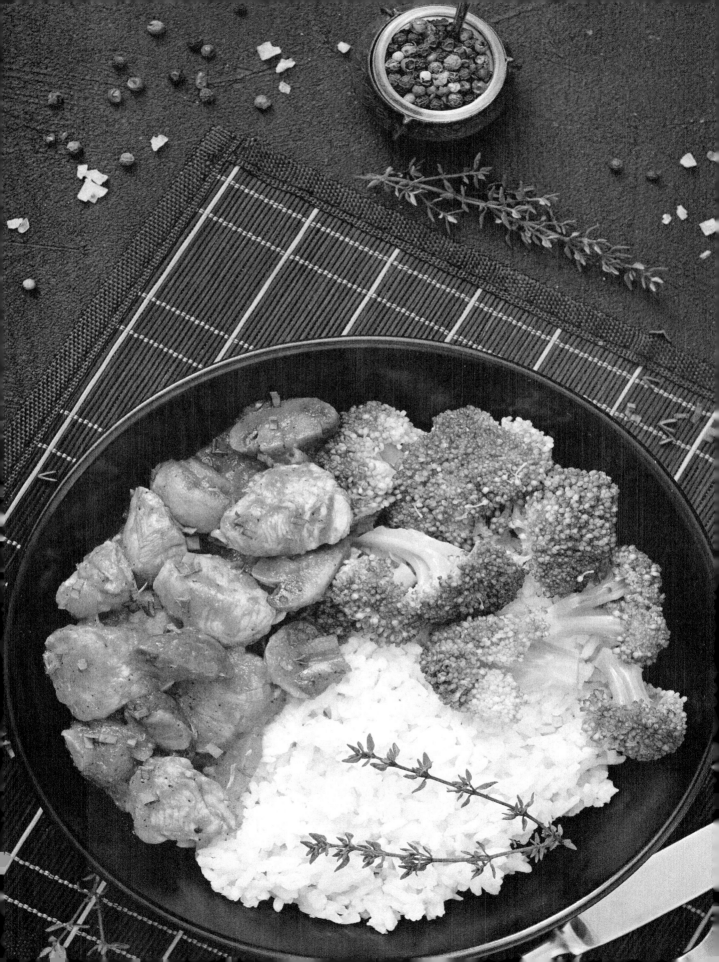

Sea Bass with Tomatoes, Olives, and Capers

 Prep Time: 10 minutes   Cooking Time: 15 minutes   Servings: 4

INGREDIENTS

4 (5-oz) sea bass fillets
1 small onion, diced
½ cup low-sodium vegetable or chicken broth
1 cup canned diced tomatoes
2 cups packed spinach
½ cup pitted and chopped Kalamata olives
2 tbsp capers, drained
2 tbsp extra-virgin olive oil
1 tsp salt
¼ tsp freshly ground black pepper

DIRECTIONS

1. Preheat the oven to 375 F.
2. Add the olive oil to a baking dish. Put the fish fillets in the dish, flipping to coat both sides with the oil.
3. Top the fish with vegetable broth, onion, spinach, tomatoes, capers, olives, salt, and pepper.
4. Cover your baking dish with aluminum foil and put it in the preheated oven. Bake within 15 minutes until the fish is cooked through.

Nutrition: Calories: 273, Fat: 12g, Carbs: 5g, Protein: 35g

Summer Ratatouille

 Prep Time: 10 minutes   Cooking Time: 25 minutes   Servings: 1

INGREDIENTS

1 red bell pepper, medium seeded and diced
1 medium red onion, peeled and diced
1 medium eggplant, about 1 pound, stemmed and diced
½ cup chopped basil
1 large tomato, diced
1 small zucchini, diced
4 cloves garlic, peeled and minced
Salt & freshly ground black pepper, as needed

DIRECTIONS

1. Put the onion in a saucepan and sauté over medium heat for 10 minutes. Add water 1 tbsp at a time to keep the onions from sticking to your pan.
2. Put in the red pepper, zucchini, eggplant, and garlic. Cook for 15 minutes, covered, stirring occasionally.
3. Stir in the basil and tomatoes, and season with salt and pepper. Serve and enjoy!

Nutrition: Calories: 64, Fat: 0.48g, Carbs: 14.32g, Protein: 2.53g

Pan-Seared Chicken with Turnip Greens

 Prep Time: 15 minutes   Cooking Time: 25 minutes   Servings: 4

INGREDIENTS

2 chicken breasts, bone-
less and skinless
1 tbsp dill seasoning
½ cup low-sodium chi-
cken broth
1 bunch of turnip greens,
thinly sliced
1 chive, chopped
4 celery stalks, including
leaves, finely chopped
1 tbsp allspice
4 cloves, minced

DIRECTIONS

1. In your small bowl, rub the seasoning all over the chicken.
2. Let the broth simmer in a large cast-iron skillet over medium heat.
3. Sauté for 5 minutes, or until the turnip greens are wilted and the onions are transparent, adding the chives, cilantro, dill allspice, cloves, and nutmeg as needed.
4. Place your chicken in the center of the pan and push the vege-tables to the edges of the pan to form a ring. 7 minutes in the oven
5. Flip, cover, and cook for another 7 to 10 minutes, or until equally browned on the second side. Place the chicken on your bed of greens and top with the pan gravy.

Nutrition: Calories: 145, Fat: 2g, Carbs: 12g, Protein: 22g

Minestrone

 Prep Time: 10 minutes   Cooking Time: 20 minutes   Servings: 6

INGREDIENTS

6 cups low-sodium
vegetable broth
2 (15-oz) cans of
low-sodium kidney
beans, drained and
rinsed
1 (15- oz) can of
diced tomatoes with
Italian seasoning
1 cup finely chopped
carrots
1 cup finely chopped
celery
Salt & freshly ground
black pepper, as nee-
ded

DIRECTIONS

1. Combine the stock, beans, and tomatoes with their juices, carrots, and celery in a large saucepan. Bring to a simmer over medium heat.
2. Cook for 15 minutes, or until the flavors meld. Remove from the heat—season with salt and pepper. Serve and enjoy!

Nutrition: Calories: 238; Fat: 1g; Carbs: 44g; Protein: 15g

Rosemary Lemon Chicken

 Prep Time: 10 minutes   Cooking Time: 20 minutes   Servings: 4

INGREDIENTS

3 garlic cloves
½ cup lemon juice
1 tsp salt
3 tbsp olive oil
1 lb. chicken breast, rinsed & patted dry
½ cup rosemary

DIRECTIONS

1. Mix the lemon juice, oil, rosemary, salt, and garlic.
2. Place the chicken breast in your baking dish. Pour the mixture over and refrigerate for 2-3 hours. Grill the chicken within 6 minutes on each side. Serve end enjoy!

Nutrition: Calories: 238, Fat: 10g, Carbs: 3g, Protein: 33g

Almond Noodles with Cauliflower

 Prep Time: 15 minutes   Cooking Time: 20 minutes   Servings: 2

INGREDIENTS

8 oz brown rice noodles
4 cups cauliflower florets
½ cup nonfat or low-fat Greek yogurt
3 tbsp almond butter
2 tbsp apple cider
2 tbsp low-sodium soy sauce
1 tbsp ground fennel

DIRECTIONS

1. Pour 6 to 8 cups of water into your medium pot and bring to a boil over medium-high heat.
2. Once boiling, add your rice noodles, then cook following package instructions—usually 4 to 5 minutes, or until soft.
3. Add the cauliflower florets to the cooking water and cook for a further minute. Drain the noodles and cauliflower and set aside.
4. Mix the Greek yogurt, almond butter, apple cider, soy sauce, and fennel in a large pot over low heat. Stir constantly and cook until smooth, 8 to 10 minutes.
5. Add the noodle and cauliflower mixture to the almond sauce. Use tongs to blend well.

Nutrition: Calories: 299, Fat: 5.28g, Carbs: 55.7g, Protein: 8.71g

Baked Halibut Steaks

 Prep Time: 5 minutes   Cooking Time: 15 minutes   Servings: 4

INGREDIENTS

4 (4-oz) halibut steaks
2 tbsp extra-virgin olive oil
1 tsp za'atar
½ tsp salt
¼ tsp freshly ground black pepper
1 lemon, cut into wedges
2 tbsp chopped fresh parsley

DIRECTIONS

1. Warm the oven to 400 F. Line a baking sheet with parchment paper.
2. Put the halibut on the prepared baking sheet. Drizzle with the oil—season both sides with the za'atar, salt, and pepper.
3. Transfer your baking sheet to the oven, and bake for 6 to 8 minutes. Flip and cook for 5 minutes until the halibut has cooked through and flakes easily with a fork. Remove from the oven.
4. Serve the halibut topped with lemon wedges and parsley.

Nutrition: Calories: 164; Fat: 8g; Carbs: 0g; Protein: 21g

Crispy Almond Chicken Breast

 Prep Time: 10 minutes   Cooking Time: 25 minutes   Servings: 4

INGREDIENTS

4 4-oz boneless, skinless chicken breasts
½ cup almond meal
½ tsp black pepper
1/8 tsp salt

DIRECTIONS

1. Preheat the oven to 350 F.
2. Combine almond meal, salt, and pepper in a resealable bag. Put each chicken breast in the bag one at a time, close the bag and shake until evenly coated. Place chicken in a glass baking dish.
3. Bake in your preheated oven until no longer pink in the middle and juices run clear, about 25 to 30 minutes. Serve with a fresh green salad if you like.

Nutrition: Calories: 222, Fat: 11g, Carbs: 3g, Protein: 28g

All Spice-Crusty Roasted Salmon

 Prep Time: 5 minutes   Cooking Time: 20 minutes   Servings: 4

INGREDIENTS

Nonstick cooking spray
½ tsp allspice
¼ tsp basil
Zest and juice of ½ lemon
¼ tsp dried Italian seasoning
1 pound salmon fillet

DIRECTIONS

1. Warm the oven to 425 F. Spray a baking sheet with nonstick cooking spray.
2. Combine allspice, basil, lemon zest and juice, and Italian seasoning in a small bowl. Stir to combine.
3. Put the salmon on your baking sheet, skin-side down. Spread the seasoning mixture evenly over the fillet.
4. Bake within 15 to 20 minutes, depending on the thickness of the fillet until the flesh flakes easily.

Nutrition: Calories: 163, Fat: 7g, Carbs:`1g, Protein: 23g

Chicken and Celery Soup

 Prep Time: 15 minutes   Cooking Time: 25 minutes   Servings: 4

INGREDIENTS

¾ pound chicken breasts, boneless, skinless, cut into 1-inch pieces
1 medium onion, sliced
1-pound beets, peeled and grated
3 medium celeries, diced
2 cups low-sodium chicken broth
1 tbsp extra-virgin olive oil
1 clove of garlic, minced
1 tsp dried tarragon
1 tsp dried dill
¼ cup chopped fresh basil
Salt and black pepper, as needed

DIRECTIONS

1. In your large Dutch oven or soup pot, heat the oil over medium-high until it begins to shimmer.
2. Whisk in the chicken, onion, and garlic and cook until the chicken is browned, 5 to 7 minutes.
3. Pour in the broth, 2 cups of water, and stir in the beets, celeries, tarragon, and dried dill until combined well.
4. Let it boil, lower the heat, cover, then simmer until the vegetables are softened, within 15 to 20 minutes. Mix in the fresh basil and drizzle with salt and black pepper to taste.

Nutrition: Calories: 207, Fat: 6g, Carbs: 20g, Protein: 21g

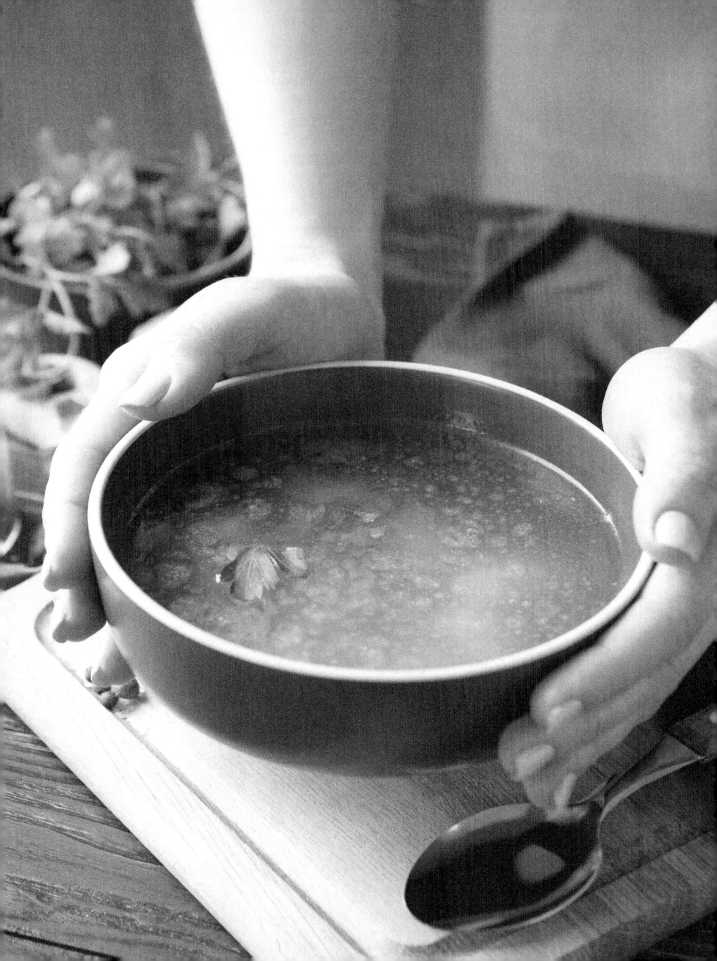

Eggplant and Chickpea Stew

 Prep Time: 15 minutes   Cooking Time: 50 minutes   Servings: 6

INGREDIENTS

1½ pounds eggplant, diced
½ tsp salt, divided
2 tbsp extra-virgin olive oil
1 onion, chopped
2 (15- oz) cans of low-sodium chickpeas, drained and rinsed
1 (28-oz) can of low-sodium diced tomatoes
2 cups water, plus more as needed
½ tsp freshly ground black pepper
Crusty bread for serving

DIRECTIONS

1. Put the eggplant in your colander, and sprinkle with ¼ teaspoon of salt. Let it rest within 10 minutes, then press to extract as much water as possible.
2. In your large pot, heat the oil over medium-high heat. Add the onion, and sauté for 3 to 5 minutes, or until browned.
3. Add the eggplant, chickpeas, and tomatoes with their juices, water, pepper, and remaining ¼ teaspoon of salt.
4. Reduce the heat to medium-low. Cover the pot, and simmer within 30 to 45 minutes, or until the eggplant is tender.
5. Open the lid and stir the mixture a couple of times as it cooks, adding more water, ½ cup at a time, to form a sauce. Remove from the heat and serve.

Nutrition: Calories: 206; Fat: 7g; Carbs: 31g; Protein: 8g

Seared Scallops

 Prep Time: 5 minutes   Cooking Time: 6 minutes   Servings: 4

INGREDIENTS

2 tbsp olive oil, divided
1½ pounds of sea scallops
2 cups chopped tomato
½ cup chopped fresh basil
¼ tsp freshly ground black pepper, divided
1/8 tsp salt
1 cup fresh corn kernels
1 cup zucchini, diced

DIRECTIONS

1. Combine tomato, basil, and 1/8 teaspoon black pepper in a medium bowl. Toss gently.
2. Heat a large skillet over high heat. Pour 1 tbsp of olive oil into your pan, swirling to coat. Pat scallops dry with paper towels. Sprinkle with salt and remaining black pepper.
3. Add scallops to your pan, and cook for 2 minutes or until browned. Then turn scallops and cook for 2 minutes more or until browned. Remove scallops and keep warm.
4. Heat the remaining olive oil in your pan. Add corn and zucchini to the pan. Sauté within 2 minutes or until lightly browned. Add to tomato mixture and toss gently.
5. Serve scallops with a spinach salad, if desired.

Nutrition: Calories: 221, Fat: 9g, Carbs: 17g, Protein: 20g

Green Pesto Pasta

 Prep Time: 5 minutes   Cooking Time: 15 minutes   Servings: 2

INGREDIENTS

4 oz spaghetti, cooked
2 cups basil leaves
2 garlic cloves
¼ cup olive oil
2 tbsp nonfat or low-fat parmesan cheese
½ tsp black pepper

DIRECTIONS

1. Add parmesan cheese, basil leaves, and garlic, and blend it well in a blender.
2. Add olive oil and pepper and blend again. Pour this pesto mixture onto pasta and serve!

Nutrition: Calories: 310, Carbs: 51g, Fat: 8g, Protein: 11g

Weeknight Fish Skillet

 Prep Time: 5 minutes   Cooking Time: 20 minutes   Servings: 4

INGREDIENTS

1 pound cod, halibut, or mahi-mahi fillets
½ tsp salt
¼ tsp freshly ground black pepper
1 tbsp extra-virgin olive oil
1 red bell pepper, cored and chopped
1 red onion, chopped
2 cups cherry tomatoes
¼ cup chopped pitted green olives

DIRECTIONS

1. Season the fillets with salt plus pepper.
2. In your large skillet, heat the oil over medium-high heat. Add the bell pepper and onion. Cook within 3 to 5 minutes, or until softened.
3. Add the tomatoes and olives. Stir for 1 to 2 minutes, or until the tomatoes soften.
4. Nestle the fillets on top of the vegetables, cover the skillet, and cook for 5 to 10 minutes until the fillets flake easily with a fork. Remove from the heat.

Nutrition: Calories: 151; Fat: 5g; Carbs: 8g; Protein: 19g

Italian Herb Turkey Cutlets

 Prep Time: 10 minutes   Cooking Time: 30 minutes   Servings: 4

INGREDIENTS

4 (4-oz) boneless, skinless turkey cutlets
3 small cloves garlic, minced
2 tbsp chopped fresh rosemary
2 tbsp chopped fresh parsley
1½ tsp chopped fresh sage
½ tsp cracked black pepper
Grated zest of 1 large lemon
1 cup low-sodium vegetable broth

DIRECTIONS

1. Preheat the oven to 375 F.
2. Mix the garlic, rosemary, parsley, sage, and pepper in a small bowl. Rub a generous amount of the herb mixture on both sides of each cutlet.
3. Place the turkey cutlets in a 9- by 13-inch baking dish, top with lemon zest, and add the vegetable broth to the dish.
4. Cover with foil, and bake within 20 to 25 minutes. Remove the foil during the last 5 minutes of baking to brown the tops of the cutlets. Remove from the oven and serve immediately.

Nutrition: Calories: 129, Fat: 2g, Carbs: 7g, Protein: 19.6g

Casserole Pizza

 Prep Time: 10 minutes   Cooking Time: 15 minutes   Servings: 6

INGREDIENTS

1 pizza crust
½ cup tomato sauce
¼ black pepper
1 cup zucchini slices
1 cup nonfat or low-fat mozzarella cheese
1 cup olives

DIRECTIONS

1. Pour and spread the tomato sauce on your pizza crust, and place the rest of the fixings on top.
2. Bake the pizza at 425 F within 12-15 minutes. When ready, remove the pizza from the oven and serve.

Nutrition: Calories: 320, Carbs: 32g, Fat: 10g, Protein: 25g

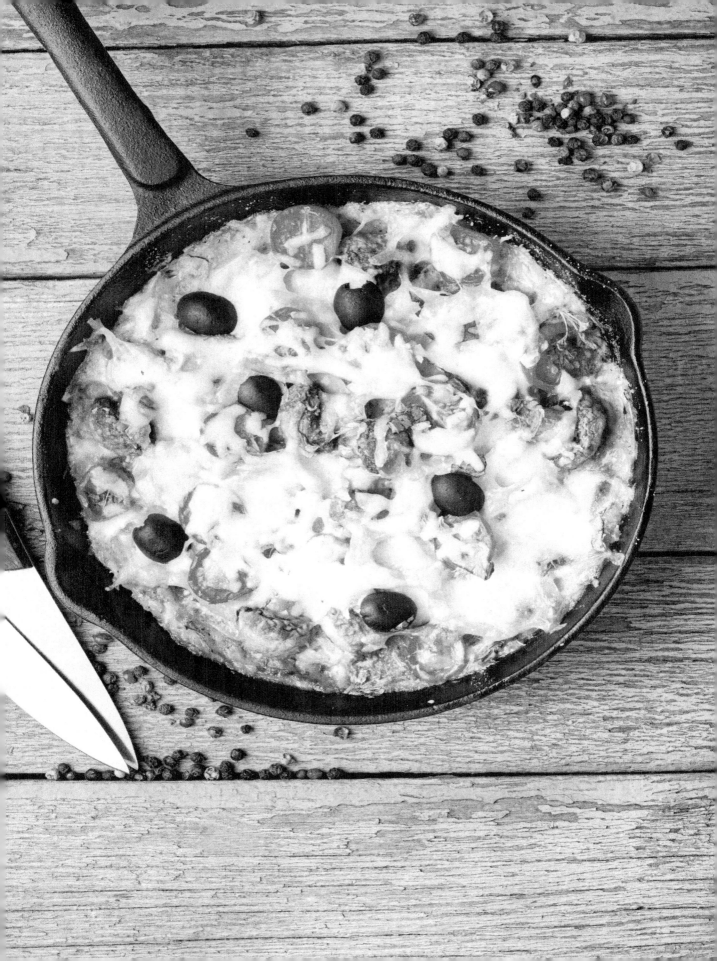

Roasted Salmon with Asparagus

 Prep Time: 5 minutes   Cooking Time: 15 minutes   Servings: 2

INGREDIENTS

2 (5-oz) salmon fillets with skin
2 tsp olive oil, + extra for drizzling
Salt & freshly ground black pepper, as needed
1 bunch asparagus, trimmed
1 tsp dried chives
1 tsp dried tarragon
Fresh lemon wedges for serving

DIRECTIONS

1. Preheat the oven to 425 F.
2. Rub salmon all over with 1 teaspoon of olive oil per fillet. Season with salt and pepper.
3. Place asparagus spears on a foil-lined baking sheet and lay the salmon fillets skin-side down on top.
4. Put your pan in the upper third of the oven and roast until the fish is just cooked through, about 12 minutes.
5. When cooked, remove from the oven, cut fillets in half crosswise, then lift flesh from the skin with your metal spatula and transfer to a plate.
6. Discard the skin, then drizzle salmon with oil, sprinkle with herbs, and serve with lemon wedges and roasted asparagus spears.

Nutrition: Calories: 353; Fat: 9g; Carbs: 5g; Protein: 34g

Stewed Chicken with Asparagus and Carrot

 Prep Time: 10 minutes   Cooking Time: 35 minutes   Servings: 10

INGREDIENTS

2 cups zucchini, diced small
2 cups cooked chicken breast, cubed
1 cup cucumber, diced
2 cups tomatoes, peeled
2 cups carrots, shredded
5 cups low sodium chicken broth
1 cup sweet corn
1 cup peas
1 cup asparagus, diced
parsley for garnishing

DIRECTIONS

1. Set a large stockpot over medium heat. Add the zucchini, chicken stock, chicken, tomatoes, cucumber, carrots, corn, asparagus, and peas.
2. Allow cooking for about half an hour over a medium flame, stirring continuously. Once done, place into a serving bowl and garnish with parsley.

Nutrition: Calories: 111, Fat: 2.5g, Carb: 13.1g, Protein: 10.1g

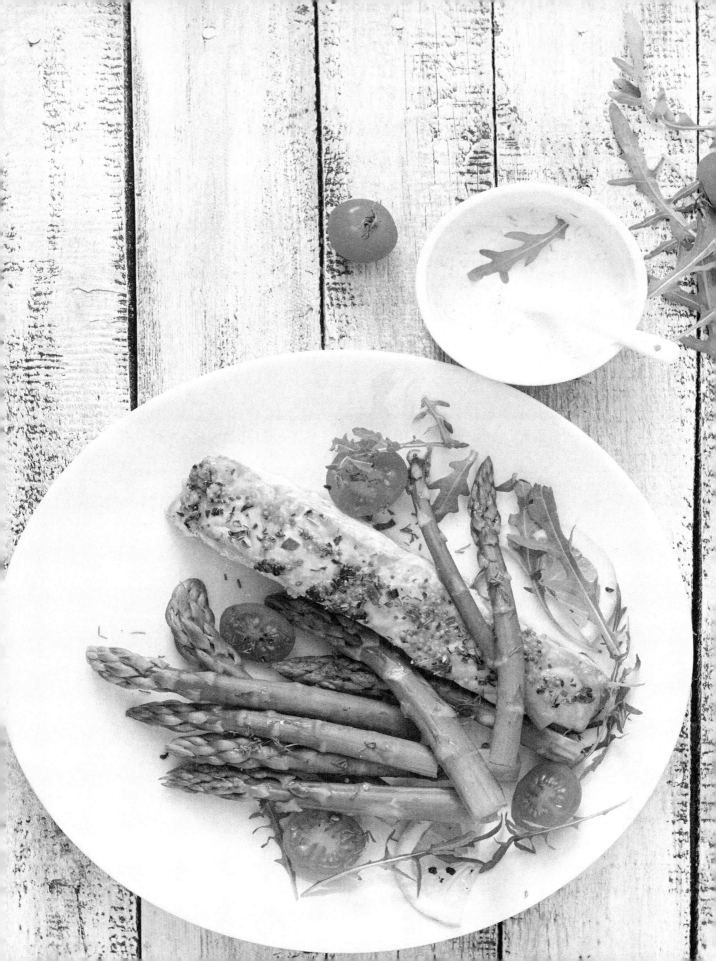

Sweet-and-Sour Trout with Chard

 Prep Time: 10 minutes   Cooking Time: 15 minutes   Servings: 4

INGREDIENTS

4 boneless trout fillets
1 tbsp extra-virgin olive oil
2 garlic cloves, minced
1 onion, chopped
2 bunches of chard, sliced
¼ cup golden raisins
1 tbsp apple cider vinegar
½ cup low sodium vegetable broth
Salt & freshly ground black pepper, as needed

DIRECTIONS

1. Preheat the oven to 375 F.
2. Season the trout with salt and pepper.
3. Heat the olive oil in your large ovenproof pan over medium-high heat. Add the onion and garlic. Sauté for 3 minutes; add the chard and sauté for another 2 minutes.
4. Add the cider vinegar, raisins, and broth to the pan—Layer the trout fillets on top. Cover your pan, then put it in the preheated oven for about 10 minutes until the trout is cooked through.

Nutrition: Calories: 231, Fat: 10g, Carbs: 13g, Protein: 24g

Buckwheat with Bow-Tie Pasta

 Prep Time: 15 minutes   Cooking Time: 35 minutes   Servings: 4

INGREDIENTS

8 oz button mushrooms, sliced
½ pound whole-grain farfalle, cooked, drained, and kept warm
2 cups low-sodium vegetable broth
1 cup buckwheat groats
1 yellow onion, large, peeled and diced small
2 tbsp finely chopped dill
Salt & freshly ground black pepper, as needed

DIRECTIONS

1. Put vegetable stock in a medium saucepan and boil over high heat. Add the buckwheat groats and bring the pot back to a boil over high heat.
2. Adjust the heat to medium and cook within 12 to 15 minutes with the lid uncovered until the groats are tender.
3. Put the onion in a large saucepan and sauté for about 15 minutes over medium heat until well browned. Pour water 1 tbsp at a time to keep the onion from sticking.
4. Add the mushrooms and cook for 5 more minutes. Remove from the heat. Add the buckwheat groats, cooked pasta, and dill. Season with salt and pepper, and serve.

Nutrition: Calories: 328, Fat: 2.07g, Carbs: 76.93g, Protein: 12.07g

Soups & Salads

Carrot Soup

 Prep Time: 10 minutes Cooking Time: 60 minutes Servings: 6

INGREDIENTS

1 tbsp avocado oil
1 onion, peeled and chopped
1-pound carrots, peeled and sliced
1 large sweet potato, peeled and diced
2 bay leaves
6 cups low-sodium chicken stock
Salt & freshly ground black pepper, as needed

DIRECTIONS

1. Heat the oil in your large saucepan over medium heat.
2. Add the onion and occasionally stir until tender but not golden, 8 to 10 minutes—season with salt and pepper.
3. Add the carrot, sweet potato, bay leaves, and 5 cups of vegetable broth. Cover the pot. Cook within 30 to 45 minutes until the vegetables are very tender.
4. Remove the bay leaves. Mix the soup in a mixer or food processor until very smooth—season with salt and pepper. Serve hot.

Nutrition: Calories: 176; Fat: 5.36 g; Carbs: 25 g; Protein: 7.5 g

---

Four-Bean Salad

 Prep Time: 10 minutes Cooking Time: 10 minutes Servings: 4

INGREDIENTS

½ cup fava beans, cooked
½ cup lima beans, cooked
½ cup white beans, cooked
½ cup black-eyed peas, cooked
1 red bell pepper, diced
1 small bunch of flat-leaf parsley, chopped
Juice of 1 lemon
Sea salt & freshly ground pepper, as needed
2 tbsp olive oil
1 tsp ground cumin

DIRECTIONS

1. Put all the fixings in a large bowl and mix well—season to taste.
2. Set aside for 30 minutes, so the flavors can come together before serving.

Nutrition: Calories: 224, Fat: 7.67g, Carbs: 30.47g, Protein: 11.25g

Creamy Pumpkin Soup

 Prep Time: 5 minutes   Cooking Time: 10 minutes   Servings: 4

INGREDIENTS

3 cups low-sodium vegetable broth, divided
7 ounces soft tofu
1 (15-oz) can of pumpkin puree
1 tbsp grated fresh ginger
½ tsp ground cinnamon
Salt & freshly ground black pepper, as needed

DIRECTIONS

1. In your blender, combine 1 cup of broth and the tofu. Process until smooth.
2. In a large saucepan, combine the tofu, remaining 2 cups of broth, the pumpkin puree, ginger, and cinnamon. Bring to a boil.
3. Reduce the heat to a simmer—Cook for 10 minutes, or until the flavors meld. Remove from the heat—season with salt and pepper.

Nutrition: Calories: 68; Fat: 2g; Carbs: 10g; Protein: 4g

Arugula Cucumber Salad

 Prep Time: 5 minutes   Cooking Time: 0 minutes   Servings: 2

INGREDIENTS

½ tsp salt
4 cucumbers
3 tbsp olive oil
6 oz arugula
2 tbsp lemon juice

DIRECTIONS

1. Mix all the fixings in a large bowl until well combined.
2. Serve and enjoy!

Nutrition: Calories: 40, Carbs: 3g, Fat: 3g, Protein: 1g

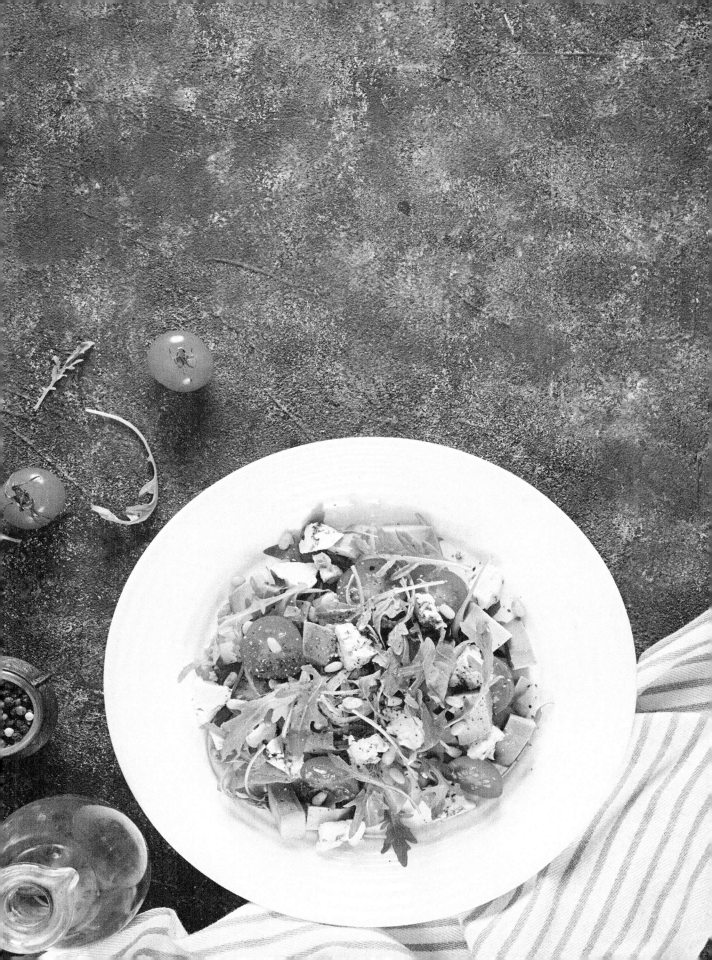

Zucchini Soup

 Prep Time: 10 minutes   Cooking Time: 20 minutes   Servings: 4

INGREDIENTS

1 tbsp olive oil
1 lb. zucchini
¼ red onion
½ cup whole wheat flour
¼ tsp salt
¼ tsp pepper
1 can low-sodium vegetable broth
1 cup dairy-free heavy cream

DIRECTIONS

1. In a saucepan, heat olive oil and sauté zucchini until tender. Add remaining ingredients to the saucepan and bring to a boil.
2. When all the vegetables are tender, transfer to a blender and blend until smooth. Pour soup into bowls, garnish with parsley and serve.

Nutrition: Calories: 60, Carbs: 10g, Fat: 1g, Protein: 4g

Avocado Salad

 Prep Time: 5 minutes   Cooking Time: 0 minutes   Servings: 2

INGREDIENTS

1 cup corn
1 cup tomatoes
1 cup cucumber
½ cup avocado
½ cup edamame
1 cup salad dressing of your choice, nonfat or low fat

DIRECTIONS

1. In a bowl, combine all fixings and mix well.
2. Serve with dressing!

Nutrition: Calories: 130, Carbs: 21g, Fat: 5g, Protein: 1g

Lemony Kale Salad

 Prep Time: 10 minutes   Cooking Time: 10 minutes   Servings: 4

INGREDIENTS

2 heads of kale, tear into pieces
Sea salt and freshly ground pepper, as needed
Juice of 1 lemon
1+ tbsp olive oil
2 cloves garlic, minced
1 cup cherry tomatoes, sliced

DIRECTIONS

1. Heat olive oil in your large skillet, then add the garlic. Cook for 1 minute, and then add the kale. Add the tomatoes after the kale wilted.
2. Cook until tomatoes are softened, then remove from heat. Put tomatoes and kale together in a bowl, and season with sea salt and freshly ground pepper.
3. Drizzle with remaining olive oil plus lemon juice, and serve.

Nutrition: Calories: 59, Fat: 3.83g, Carbs: 5.95g, Protein: 2g

---

Spinach Soup

 Prep Time: 10 minutes   Cooking Time: 20 minutes   Servings: 4

INGREDIENTS

1 tbsp olive oil
1 lb. spinach
¼ red onion
½ cup all-purpose flour
¼ tsp salt
¼ tsp pepper
1 can vegetable broth
1 cup dairy-free heavy cream

DIRECTIONS

1. In a saucepan, heat olive oil and sauté spinach until tender. Add remaining ingredients to the saucepan and bring to a boil.
2. When all the vegetables are tender, transfer to a blender and blend until smooth. Pour soup into bowls, garnish with parsley and serve.

Nutrition: Calories: 50, Carbs: 5g, Fat: 3g, Protein: 4g

Cantaloupe Salad

 Prep Time: 5 minutes   Cooking Time: 0 minutes   Servings: 2

INGREDIENTS

2 cups watermelon
1 cup cantaloupe
1 tbsp honey
1 tbsp mint
1 tsp arugula leaves
½ cup nonfat or low-fat feta cheese

DIRECTIONS

1. In a bowl, combine all fixings and mix well.
2. Serve with dressing!

Nutrition: Calories: 53, Carbs: 11g, Fat: 0g, Protein: 1g

Tomato Basil Soup

 Prep Time: 5 minutes   Cooking Time: 10 minutes   Servings: 4

INGREDIENTS

1 tsp olive oil
1 cup chopped onion
4 garlic cloves, minced
7 cups chopped fresh tomatoes (aim for a mix of large, cherry, grape, and heirloom)
½ cup chopped fresh basil leaves
1/8 tsp salt
1 tsp freshly ground black pepper

DIRECTIONS

1. Heat the olive oil in your medium saucepan over medium heat. Add the onion and garlic and cook for 1 to 2 minutes.
2. Put the tomatoes and continue to cook, stirring every few minutes until the tomatoes have broken down and are soft. Remove and add the basil, salt, and pepper.
3. Purée in a blender or use an immersion blender until smooth. Serve immediately.

Nutrition: Calories: 169; Fats: 4g; Carbs: 33g; Protein: 7g

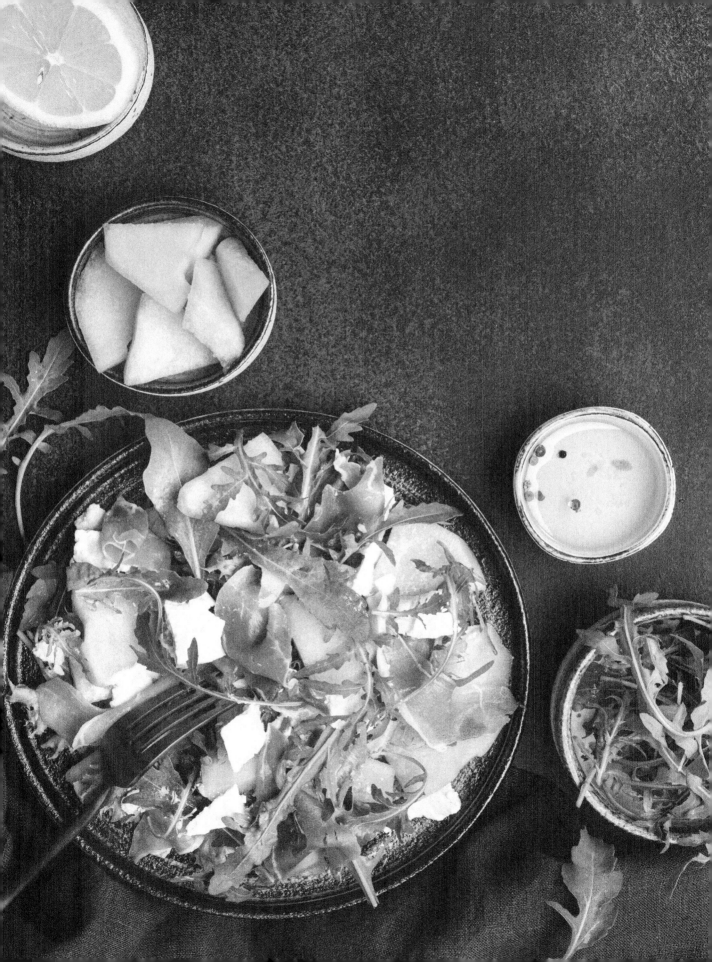

Asparagus Soup

 Prep Time: 10 minutes   Cooking Time: 35 minutes   Servings: 6

INGREDIENTS

2 pounds fresh aspa-
ragus, trimmed & cut
into ½-inch pieces
1 large yellow onion,
peeled and diced
4 cups low-sodium
vegetable broth
2 tsp thyme
1 tbsp. minced tarra-
gon
Salt & freshly ground
black pepper to taste

DIRECTIONS

1. Prepare a large stockpot, put the onion, and sauté over medium heat for 10 minutes. Pour 1 to 2 tbsp of water at a time to prevent the onion from sticking to the pot.
2. Add the thyme, tarragon, vegetable stock, and asparagus and cook on medium-low heat for 20 to 25 minutes, until the asparagus is soft.
3. Use your immersion blender or a blender to puree the soup in batches. Close the lid and cover with a towel. Salt and pepper to taste, then serve!

Nutrition: Calories: 70, Fat: 0.52g, Carbs: 14.37g, Protein: 5.62g

---

Kentucky Salad

 Prep Time: 10 minutes   Cooking Time: 5-7 minutes   Servings: 2

INGREDIENTS

½ head of lettuce,
cut into bite-size
pieces
2 tbsp berries
½ grapefruit
2 tbsp raspberry vine-
gar
Salt & pepper, as
needed
5 tbsp olive oil
4 oz turkey breast, cut
into strips

DIRECTIONS

1. Cut the top and bottom off the grapefruit, and carefully cut away the skin. Cut the grapefruit into segments.
2. Mix the lettuce, berries, and grapefruit in your large bowl until well combined.
3. Mix the vinegar, salt, pepper, and 3 tbsp of oil. Pour this mixture over your salad and toss well.
4. Heat the remaining oil in a pan. Fry the turkey strips for 5 to 7 minutes until golden and cooked through. Season with salt and pepper.
5. Place the turkey on top of your salad and serve immediately.

Nutrition: Calories: 423, Carbs: 35g, Fat: 10g, Protein: 42g

Cucumber Soup

 Prep Time: 10 minutes   Cooking Time: 20 minutes   Servings: 4

INGREDIENTS

1 tbsp olive oil
1 lb. cucumber
¼ red onion
½ cup all-purpose flour
¼ tsp salt
¼ tsp pepper
1 can low-sodium vege-
table broth
1 cup dairy-free heavy
cream

DIRECTIONS

1. In a saucepan, heat olive oil and sauté onion until tender. Add remaining ingredients to the saucepan and bring to a boil.
2. When all the vegetables are tender, transfer to a blender and blend
until smooth. Pour soup into bowls, garnish with parsley and serve.

Nutrition: Calories: 128, Carbs: 5g, Fat: 0g, Protein: 3g

Apple & Raisin Salad

 Prep Time: 10 minutes   Cooking Time: 0 minutes   Servings: 6

INGREDIENTS

2 tbsp olive oil
2 tsp freshly squeezed
lemon juice
Pinch of salt
4 apples, sliced into
strips
¾ cup pecans, toa-
sted and chopped
½ cup fresh cilantro
leaves
¼ cup dried cranber-
ries
¼ cup golden raisins

DIRECTIONS

1. Add all the fixings to a bowl, and toss until fully combined.
2. Serve and enjoy!

Nutrition: Calories: 108, Carbs: 26g, Fat: 2g, Protein: 1g

Squash and Peach Soup with Mint

 Prep Time: 10 minutes   Cooking Time: 30 minutes   Servings: 4

INGREDIENTS

1 medium zucchini, peeled and diced small
1 large winter squash, acorn, or butternut, peeled, halved, seeded, and cut into ½-inch dice (about 6 cups)
2 peaches, peeled, cored, and diced
1 cup unsweetened almond butter
3 cups low-sodium vegetable broth
Pinch of mint
Salt to taste

DIRECTIONS

1. Add the zucchini to a large saucepan and sauté over medium heat for 10 minutes or until the zucchini is browned.
2. Pour water 1 to 2 tbsp at a time to keep your onion from sticking to the pan. Stir in the squash, peaches, almond butter, vegetable stock, and mint, and bring to a boil over high heat.
3. Adjust the heat down to medium and simmer, covered, for about 20 minutes, or until the squash is softened.
4. Pulse the soup in a food processor, and cover with a towel. If necessary, return the soup to the pot to reheat. Sprinkle with salt to taste.

Nutrition: Calories: 151, Fat: 0.95g, Carbs: 35.7g, Protein: 3.93g

---

Sweetcorn Soup

 Prep Time: 10 minutes   Cooking Time: 20 minutes   Servings: 4

INGREDIENTS

1 tbsp olive oil
1 lb. sweetcorn
¼ red onion
½ cup all-purpose flour
¼ tsp salt
¼ tsp pepper
1 can low-sodium vegetable broth
1 cup dairy-free heavy cream

DIRECTIONS

1. In a saucepan, heat olive oil and sauté onion until tender. Add remaining ingredients to the saucepan and bring to a boil.
2. When all the vegetables are tender, transfer to a blender and blend until smooth. Pour soup into bowls, garnish with parsley and serve.

Nutrition: Calories: 168, Carbs: 16g, Fat: 8g, Protein: 6g

Fruit Salad

 Prep Time: 10 minutes   Cooking Time: 0 minutes   Servings: 2

INGREDIENTS

1 cup mixed berries
3 tbsp nonfat or low-fat Greek yogurt, unsweetened
½ tbsp chia seeds
½ vanilla bean scraped
1 sage leaf, cut into small pieces

DIRECTIONS

1. Add the berries to your large bowl and mix in the chopped sage.
2. In a small bowl, mix the Greek yogurt, chia seeds, and scraped vanilla until well mixed, then set aside for 5 minutes.
3. Add the yogurt mixture to the berries and mix well. Chill in the fridge before serving.

Nutrition: Calories: 151; Fat: 2.3 g; Carbs: 6 g; Protein: 8 g

---

Coconut-Black Bean Soup

 Prep Time: 10 minutes   Cooking Time: 30 minutes   Servings: 6

INGREDIENTS

4 cups canned black beans, drained, rinsed
2 cups diced tomatoes
2 cups coconut milk
1 cup low-sodium vegetable broth
1 cup chopped green onions
2 cloves garlic, minced
1 tbsp ground turmeric
1 tbsp ground cumin
1 tbsp ground ginger
1 pinch salt

DIRECTIONS

1. In your saucepan, mix all the ingredients and bring to a gentle boil. Lower heat and simmer, covered, for about 30 minutes.
2. Remove and serve hot cooked rice if you like.

Nutrition: Calories: 110, Carbs: 60g, Fat: 2g, Protein: 6g

Quinoa Salad

 Prep Time: 10 minutes   Cooking Time: 20 minutes   Servings: 4

INGREDIENTS

1 cup quinoa
½ cup cranberries
3 tsp olive oil
½ onion
1 bunch of kale
2 tsp salt
1 ½ tsp black pepper
1 cup nonfat or low-fat feta cheese
½ cup almonds
3 tsp lemon juice

DIRECTIONS

1. Cook the quinoa for 15 minutes in boiling salted water. Drain in a sieve, add the cranberries, cover, and set aside.
2. Heat 1 ½ tsp oil and sauté the onion. Add the kale and cook for 5 minutes—season with salt.
3. Add the kale to quinoa, feta and almonds, and lemon juice. Serve and enjoy!

Nutrition: Calories: 150, Carbs: 23g, Fat: 2g, Protein: 4g

Lentil and Veggie Soup

 Prep Time: 10 minutes   Cooking Time: 40 minutes   Servings: 4

INGREDIENTS

2 tbsp extra-virgin olive oil
1 medium onion, chopped
2 carrots, chopped
1 cup dried brown lentils
1 (28-oz) can of low-sodium diced tomatoes
4 cups water
Juice of 1 lemon
Salt & freshly ground black pepper, as needed

DIRECTIONS

1. In your large saucepan, heat the oil over medium-high heat. Add the onion and carrots. Sauté for 3 to 5 minutes, or until just starting to soften.
2. Add your lentils, tomatoes with their juices, and water. Bring to a boil.
3. Reduce the heat to a simmer—Cook within 25 to 30 minutes, or until the lentils are tender. Remove from the heat.
4. Remove 2 cups from the saucepan, process it in a blender, and return it to the saucepan.
5. Add the lemon juice—season with salt and pepper. Serve and enjoy!

Nutrition: Calories: 287; Fat: 8g; Carbs: 44g; Protein: 14g

Baked Beet Salad

 Prep Time: 10 minutes　　 Cooking Time: 35 minutes　　 Servings: 4

INGREDIENTS

3 or 4 medium beets
1 (8-oz) bag arugula
¼ cup balsamic vinaigrette
¼ cup chopped almonds

DIRECTIONS

1. Preheat the oven to 350 F.
2. Wash the beets well. Wrap them in aluminum foil.
3. Transfer the beets to the oven, and bake for 25 to 35 minutes, depending on the size of the beets, or until easily pierced with a fork. Remove from the oven. Let cool until easy to handle.
4. Slide the skins off your beets and discard them using your hands. Cut the beets into wedges.
5. Put the beets in a large bowl with the arugula. Drizzle the vinaigrette over the beets, and toss gently. Serve the salad topped with the almonds.

Nutrition: Calories: 60, Carbs: 14g, Fat: 0g, Protein: 2g

Creamy Tomato Soup

 Prep Time: 10 minutes　　 Cooking Time: 2 minutes　　 Servings: 1

INGREDIENTS

¾ cup no-salt canned tomato puree
¼ cup low-sodium chicken broth
1 tbsp nonfat or low-fat cream cheese

DIRECTIONS

1. Whisk the puree with the broth and cream cheese in a big heat-proof mug.
2. Microwave using the high setting, occasionally stirring until thoroughly heated and creamy, within 2 minutes. Serve and enjoy!

Nutrition: Calories: 105, Fat: 2.7g, Carbs: 18.3g, Protein: 5.1g

Caprese Salad

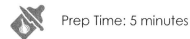 Prep Time: 5 minutes   Cooking Time: 5 minutes   Servings: 2

INGREDIENTS

3 cups tomatoes
2 oz nonfat or low-fat
mozzarella cheese
2 tbsp basil
1 tbsp olive oil

DIRECTIONS

1. In your bowl, combine all ingredients and mix well.
2. Serve with dressing, and enjoy!

Nutrition: Calories: 50, Carbs: 7g, Fat: 8g, Protein: 5g

Corn Salad

 Prep Time: 5 minutes   Cooking Time: 0 minutes   Servings: 2

INGREDIENTS

1 cup corn
1 cup cucumber
1 cup tomatoes
¼ cup avocado
1 tbsp lime juice
½ cup nonfat or low-
fat Greek yogurt
1 cup nonfat or low-
fat salad dressing of
your choice

DIRECTIONS

1. In your bowl, combine all ingredients and mix well.
2. Serve with dressing!

Nutrition: Calories: 80, Carbs: 19g, Fat: 1g, Protein: 2g

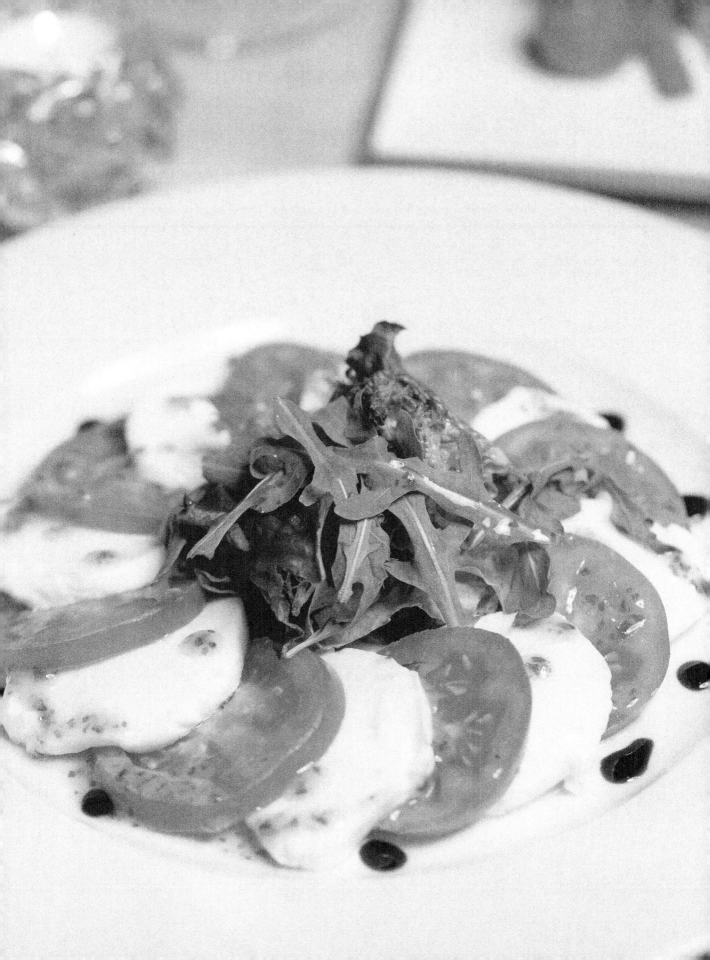

Carrot Apple Salad

 Prep Time: 10 minutes   Cooking Time: 0 minutes   Servings: 4

INGREDIENTS

2 large Granny Smith apples, sliced into matchsticks (about 1½ cups)
2 large carrots, cut into matchsticks (about 1½ cups)
1 cup nonfat or low-fat plain Greek yogurt
¼ cup raisins
1 tsp ground cinnamon
¼ tsp ground ginger

DIRECTIONS

1. Mix the apples and carrots into the y in a medium bowl, and then stir in the remaining ingredients.
2. Let it sit within 30 minutes before serving.

Nutrition: Calories: 117, Fat: 0.7g, Carbs: 26g, Protein: 6g

Parsnip Soup

 Prep Time: 10 minutes   Cooking Time: 20 minutes   Servings: 4

INGREDIENTS

1 tbsp olive oil
1 cup parsnip
¼ red onion
½ cup all-purpose flour
¼ tsp salt
¼ tsp pepper
1 can low-sodium vegetable broth
1 cup dairy-free heavy cream

DIRECTIONS

1. In a saucepan, heat olive oil and sauté parsnip until tender. Add remaining ingredients to the saucepan and bring to a boil.
2. When all the vegetables are tender, transfer to a blender and blend until smooth. Pour soup into bowls, garnish with parsley and serve.

Nutrition: Calories: 233, Carbs: 30g, Fat: 10g, Protein: 6g

Butternut Squash Salad

 Prep Time: 5 minutes   Cooking Time: 0 minutes   Servings: 2

INGREDIENTS

3 cups butternut squash
1 cup cooked couscous
2 cups kale leaves
2 tbsp cranberries
2 oz nonfat or low-fat
goat cheese
1 cup nonfat or low-fat
salad dressing of your
choice

DIRECTIONS

1. In your bowl, combine all ingredients and mix well. Serve with dressing!

Nutrition: Calories: 45, Carbs: 11g, Fat: 0g, Protein: 1g

Leek and Pear Soup with Fennel and Spinach

 Prep Time: 15 minutes   Cooking Time: 15 minutes   Servings: 4-6

INGREDIENTS

2 leeks, white part
only, sliced
1 fennel bulb, cut into
¼-inch-thick slices
2 tbsp extra-virgin
olive oil
2 pears, peeled,
cored, and cut into
½-inch cubes
¼ tsp freshly ground
black pepper
1 tsp salt
2 cups packed spinach or arugula
½ cup cashews
3 cups water or
low-sodium vegetable broth

DIRECTIONS

1. Add olive oil into a large Dutch oven or skillet, and heat over high heat. Place the leeks and fennel into the oven and sauté for 5 minutes.
2. Stir in the pears, salt, and pepper. Sauté for another 3 minutes.
3. Add the cashews, pour in water, and bring the soup to a boil. Lower the heat to simmer and cook for 5 minutes, partially covered. Add the spinach and stir well.
4. In a blender, pour the soup, working in batches if necessary, and purée the soup until smooth.

Nutrition: Calories: 111, Fat: 5g, Carbs: 9g, Protein: 9g

Cauliflower Soup

 Prep Time: 10 minutes   Cooking Time: 25 minutes   Servings: 6

INGREDIENTS

3 large leeks (white parts only), sliced and rinsed
4 cups cauliflower florets (from about 2 large heads)
4½ cups vegetable broth, low-sodium, + more as needed
3 tbsp apple cider
1 tsp tarragon, minced
5 cloves garlic, minced
Salt & freshly ground black pepper to taste

DIRECTIONS

1. Add the leeks to a large saucepan and sauté over medium heat for 10 minutes. Pour in water 1 to 2 tbsp at a time to keep the leeks from sticking to the pan.
2. Stir in the tarragon, cook within another minute, and stir in the cauliflower, vegetable stock, and apple cider.
3. Let it boil over high heat, turn the heat down to medium, and simmer, covered, until the cauliflower is softened, within 10 minutes.
4. Process the soup in your food processor, and cover with a towel. Return the soup to your pot and sprinkle with salt and pepper to taste.

Nutrition: Calories: 87, Fat: 0.97g, Carbs: 16.47g, Protein: 5.44g

---

Chickpea Salad with Tuna

 Prep Time: 10 minutes   Cooking Time: 0 minutes   Servings: 4

INGREDIENTS

1 English cucumber, chopped
1 (15-oz) can of chickpeas, drained & rinsed
2 (5-oz) cans of water-packed tuna, drained
½ red onion, sliced
¼ cup nonfat or low-fat salad dressing of your choice

DIRECTIONS

1. Toss together the cucumber, chickpeas, tuna, and onion in your large bowl.
2. Drizzle with your vinaigrette, and toss to combine. Serve at room temperature or cold.

Nutrition: Calories: 234; Fat: 11g; Carbs: 18g; Protein: 16g

Snacks & Appetizers

Quinoa Energy Balls

 Prep Time: 20 minutes

 Cooking Time: 0 minutes

 Servings: 24 balls

INGREDIENTS

¾ cup honey
1 cup quinoa
½ cup natural almond butter
Flax seeds for garnish

DIRECTIONS

1. Mix the honey, quinoa, and almond butter in a food processor and process until very finely chopped. Roll into 24 balls.
2. Garnish with flax seeds, if desired. Serve and enjoy!

Nutrition: Calories: 60; Fat: 0.6g; Carbs: 13.3g; Protein: 1.1g

---

Oat Nuggets

 Prep Time: 10 minutes

 Cooking Time: 0 minutes

 Servings: 30 nuggets

INGREDIENTS

1 cup rolled oats
¾ cup pecan nuts, chopped
½ cup almond butter
½ cup ground chia seeds
¼ cup organic honey
¼ cup golden raisins

DIRECTIONS

1. In your medium-sized mixing bowl, add the rolled oats, chopped pecan nuts, almond butter, ground chia seeds, organic honey, and golden raisins, and mix to incorporate.
2. Place your bowl in the fridge for 10 to 20 minutes for the contents to firm up. Roll into 30 balls. Serve and enjoy!

Nutrition: Calories: 174; Fat: 10g; Carbs: 17g; Protein: 5g

Guacamole with Jicama

 Prep Time: 5 minutes   Cooking Time: 0 minutes   Servings: 4

INGREDIENTS

1 avocado, cut into cubes
Juice of ½ lime
2 tbsp finely chopped shallots
2 tbsp chopped fresh parsley
1 garlic clove, minced
¼ tsp basil
1 cup sliced jicama

DIRECTIONS

1. Combine the avocado, lime juice, shallots, parsley, garlic, and salt in your small bowl. Mash lightly with a fork.
2. Serve with the jicama for dipping.

Nutrition: Calories: 73, Fat: 5g, Carbs: 8g, Protein: 1g

Taro Chips

 Prep Time: 10 minutes   Cooking Time: 20 minutes   Servings: 4

INGREDIENTS

1 pound taro peeled
1 tsp olive oil
A pinch of salt
A pinch of pepper

DIRECTIONS

1. Slice the taro lengthwise; place the taro slices on paper-lined baking sheets and brush with olive oil.
2. Season with sea salt and pepper and bake at 400 F for about 20 minutes or until crisp.

Nutrition: Calories: 137 Fat: 1.4 g; Carbs: 25.3 g; Protein: 1.7 g

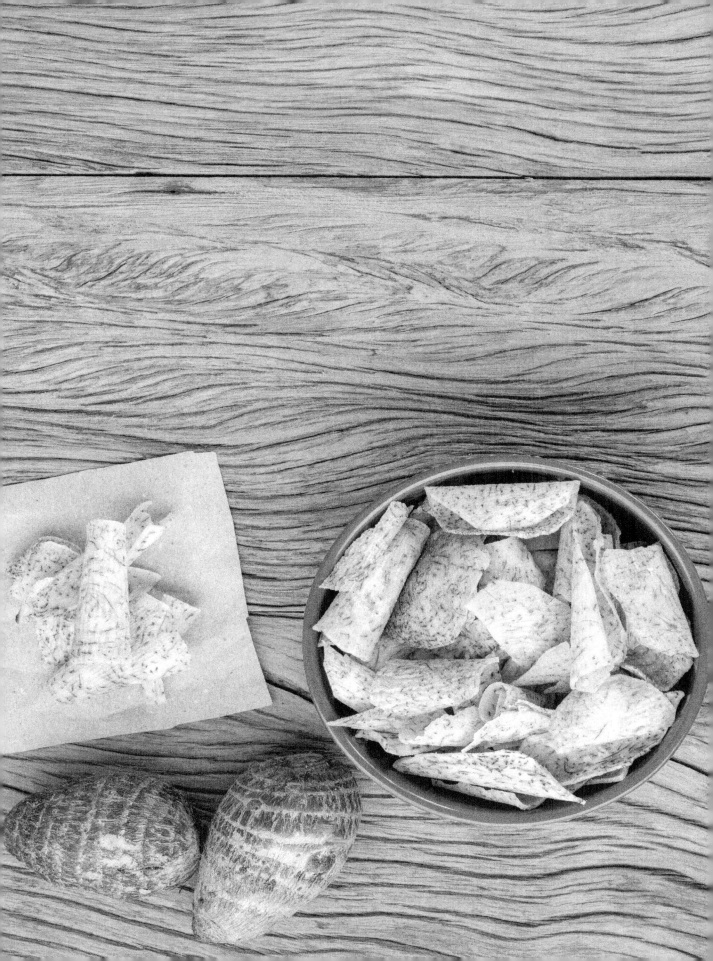

Amaranth Pop Corns

 Prep Time: 5 minutes   Cooking Time: 10 minutes   Servings: 2

INGREDIENTS

1/2 cup amaranth seeds
1 tsp olive oil
1 tsp cinnamon
½ tsp sea salt

DIRECTIONS

1. Heat olive oil in your pot set over high heat; add the amaranth seeds and cook until they start popping. Cover the pot and let all seeds pop.
2. Serve sprinkled with cinnamon and sea salt.

Nutrition: Calories: 205 Fat: 5.5 g; Carbs: 28.1 g; Protein: 7.1 g

---

Roasted Sweet Potato Fries

 Prep Time: 10 minutes   Cooking Time: 35 minutes   Servings: 4

INGREDIENTS

2 large sweet potatoes, cut into thin fries
2 tbsp extra-virgin olive oil
1 ½ garlic powder
½ tsp salt
Pinch ground cayenne pepper

DIRECTIONS

1. Warm the oven to 425 F. Line a baking sheet with parchment paper.
2. Toss together the sweet potatoes, oil, garlic powder, salt, and cayenne in a large bowl.
3. Spread your sweet potatoes out in an even layer on the prepared baking sheet.
4. Transfer your baking sheet to the oven, and bake, flipping once, for 30 to 35 minutes, or until the sweet potatoes are crisp. Remove from the oven.

Nutrition: Calories: 123; Fat: 7g; Carbs: 15g; Protein: 1g

Spinach Balls

 Prep Time: 10 minutes   Cooking Time: 15-20 minutes   Servings: 15 balls

INGREDIENTS

1 ½ tbsp olive oil
1 cup breadcrumbs
1 ½ tbsp nonfat or low-fat yogurt
2 tbsp green onion
1 10-oz package of spinach
1 egg
1 cup nonfat or low-fat cheese

DIRECTIONS

1. Mix all of the fixings in a bowl, and form them into balls.
2. Bake at 350 F for 15-20 minutes, let it cool, and serve.

Nutrition: Calories: 74, Carbs: 5g, Fat: 5g, Protein: 3g

Gingerbread Balls

 Prep Time: 10 minutes   Cooking Time: 0 minutes   Servings: 10 balls

INGREDIENTS

½ cup gluten-free rolled oats
¼ cup all-purpose flour
½ tbsp ground cinnamon
½ tsp ground ginger
¼ tsp ground nutmeg
¼ tsp pure vanilla extract
1 cup figs, pitted and chopped
1-½ tbsp powdered sweetener

DIRECTIONS

1. Put the oatmeal, all-purpose flour, cinnamon, ginger, nutmeg, and vanilla extract in a mixer.
2. Stir well until smooth. Mix the dates in batches until smooth paste forms. Form 1-inch balls and roll in the powdered sweetener. Let it chill before serving.

Nutrition: Calories: 40; Fat: 0.4g; Carbs: 8.4g; Protein: 1.1g

Zucchini Chips

 Prep Time: 5 minutes   Cooking Time: 10 minutes   Servings: 4

INGREDIENTS

2 medium zucchinis, cut into ¼-inch slices
½ cup seasoned panko bread crumbs
1/8 tsp ground black pepper
2 tbsp grated nonfat or low-fat Parmesan cheese
2 egg whites

DIRECTIONS

1. Preheat the oven to 245 F.
2. Mix breadcrumbs, pepper, and Parmesan cheese in a small bowl. Put the egg whites in another dish.
3. Dip the zucchinis into the egg whites, then coat them with breadcrumbs. Place them on a greased baking sheet.
4. Bake in the oven within 5 minutes, then flip them around and bake another 5 to 10 minutes. Serve and enjoy!

Nutrition: Calories: 127; Fat: 4g; Carbs: 14.2g; Protein: 9.6g

---

Cucumber, Jicama, & Pineapple Sticks

 Prep Time: 10 minutes   Cooking Time: 0 minutes   Servings: 2

INGREDIENTS

6 spears of cucumber
6 spears of very ripe pineapple
6 spears jicama
1 tsp seasoning of your choice
2 lime wedges

DIRECTIONS

1. In a bowl, mix cucumber, pineapple, jicama, lime juice, and seasoning until well mixed.
2. Serve garnished with lime wedges.

Nutrition: Calories: 17; Fat: 0 g; Carbs: 4.3 g; Protein: 0 g

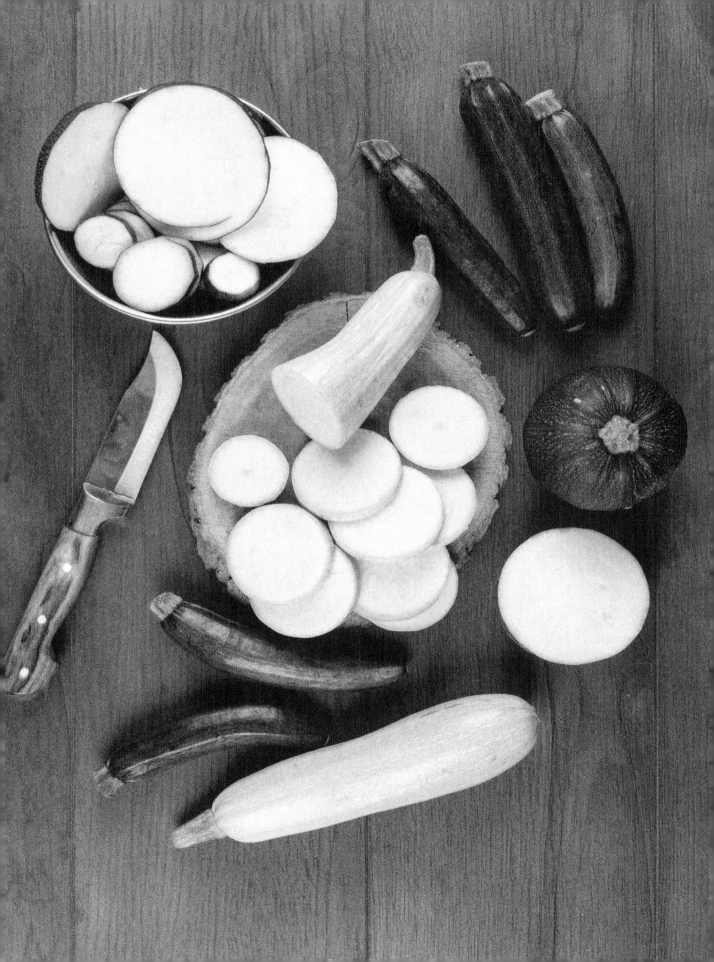

Baked Apples

 Prep Time: 10 minutes   Cooking Time: 50 minutes   Servings: 2

INGREDIENTS

½ tsp cinnamon
1 tsp olive oil
1 tbsp rolled oats
2 tsp organic honey
2 apples

DIRECTIONS

1. Preheat the oven to 325 F.
2. In a bowl, mix honey, cinnamon, oats, and oil
3. Stuff into cored apples and bake for 40-50 minutes. Remove and serve.

Nutrition: Calories: 81, Carbs: 13g, Fat: 4g, Protein: 0g

Turmeric Cashew Nut Balls

 Prep Time: 10 minutes   Cooking Time: 0 minutes   Servings: 12 balls

INGREDIENTS

1 cup raw cashews
1 1/2 cup shredded coconut
1 tbsp raw honey
3 tsp ground turmeric
1 tsp cinnamon
1 tsp ground ginger
1 tsp black pepper
1/2 tsp sea salt

DIRECTIONS

1. In a food processor, process coconut until almost oily; add the rest of the ingredients and process until cashews are finely chopped.
2. Press the mixture into bite-sized balls and arrange them on a baking tray.
3. Refrigerate until firm before serving.

Nutrition: Calories: 131; Fat: 10 g; Carbs: 7.3 g; Protein: 2.5 g

Chunky Black-Bean Dip

 Prep Time: 10 minutes   Cooking Time: 0 minutes   Servings: 6-8

INGREDIENTS

1 (15-oz) can of black beans, drained, with liquid
reserved
½ (7-oz) can of chipotle
peppers in adobo sauce
¼ cup nonfat or low-fat
plain Greek yogurt
Freshly ground black pep-
per, as needed

DIRECTIONS

1. Combine beans, peppers, and yogurt in a food processor or blender and process until smooth. Add some of the bean liquid, 1 tablespoon at a time, for a thinner consistency.
2. Season it with black pepper, and serve.

Nutrition: Calories: 70; Fat: 1g; Carbs: 11g; Protein: 5g

Crispy Potato Skins

 Prep Time: 5 minutes   Cooking Time: 19 minutes   Servings: 2

INGREDIENTS

2 russet potatoes
Cooking spray
1 tsp dried rosemary
1/8 tsp freshly ground
black pepper

DIRECTIONS

1. Preheat the oven to 375 F.
2. Wash your potatoes and pierce them several times with a fork. Place on a plate. Cook on full power in the microwave for 5 minutes.
3. Turn over, and continue to cook for 3 to 4 minutes more, or until soft.
4. Carefully cut the potatoes in half and scoop out the pulp, leaving about 1/8 inch of potato flesh attached to the skin. Save the pulp for another use.
5. Spray the inside of each potato with cooking spray. Press in the rose-mary and pepper.
6. Place the skins on a baking sheet and bake in preheated oven for 5 to 10 minutes until slightly browned and crispy. Serve immediately.

Nutrition: Calories: 114; Fat: 0g; Carbs: 27g; Protein: 3g

Cucumber Chips

 Prep Time: 10 minutes
 Cooking Time: 20 minutes
 Servings: 2

INGREDIENTS

1 lb. cucumber
1 tsp salt
1 tbsp olive oil

DIRECTIONS

1. Preheat the oven to 425 F.
2. In a bowl, toss everything with olive oil and salt.
3. Spread everything onto a prepared baking sheet. Bake for 8-10 minutes or until crisp. Serve and enjoy!

Nutrition: Calories: 45, Fat: 2g, Carbs: 8g, Protein: 1g

Roasted Lentil Snack Mix

 Prep Time: 5 minutes
 Cooking Time: 25 minutes
 Servings: 4

INGREDIENTS

1 cup dried red lentils
1 cup whole unsalted shelled pistachios
½ cup unsalted shelled sunflower seeds
½ cup dried cherries

DIRECTIONS

1. Cover the lentils with water in your bowl, soak for 1 hour, and drain them well.
2. Warm the oven to 350 F. Transfer the lentils to a clean kitchen towel and dab gently. Set aside for about 10 minutes to dry.
3. Spread the lentils out on a large baking sheet.
4. Transfer your baking sheet to the oven, and bake, stirring once or twice, for 20 to 25 minutes, or until the lentils are crisp.
5. Remove from the oven. Let cool to room temperature. Transfer to a large bowl.
6. Add the pistachios, sunflower seeds, and cherries. Toss to combine. Let it cool, and serve.

Nutrition: Calories: 125, Fat: 6g, Carbs: 16g, Protein: 3g

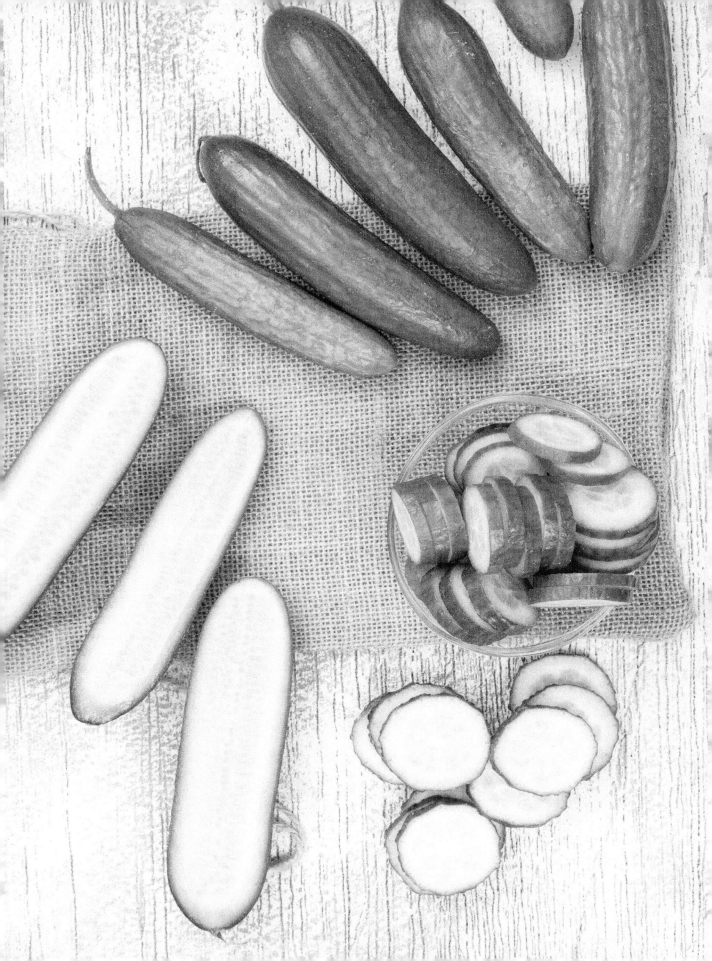

Vegetable Chips with Rosemary Salt

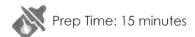 Prep Time: 15 minutes   Cooking Time: 50 minutes   Servings: 4

INGREDIENTS

Olive oil cooking spray
2 medium beets, peeled and sliced
1 medium zucchini, sliced
1 medium sweet potato, sliced
1 small rutabaga, peeled and sliced
½ tsp salt, plus more to sweat the vegetables
¼ tsp dried rosemary

DIRECTIONS

1. Preheat the oven to 300 F. Spray a baking sheet with cooking spray. Line a plate with paper towels.
2. Lay the beets, zucchini, sweet potato, and rutabaga in a single layer on a paper towel. Lightly salt, and let sit for 10 minutes.
3. Cover the vegetables with another paper towel, and blot away any moisture on top. Arrange the vegetables on your prepared baking sheet, and spray with cooking spray.
4. Transfer the baking sheet to the oven, and cook for 30 to 40 minutes, or until the vegetables have browned.
5. Flip the vegetables, and cook for 10 minutes, or until crisp. Remove from the oven. Transfer to the prepared plate to drain any excess oil.
6. In your small bowl, mix the salt and rosemary. Lightly season the chips with the rosemary salt.

Nutrition: Calories: 72; fat: 0g; Carbs: 16g; Protein: 2g

Squash Chips

 Prep Time: 10 minutes   Cooking Time: 0 minutes   Servings: 2

INGREDIENTS

1 lb. squash, sliced thinly
1 tsp salt
1 tbsp olive oil

DIRECTIONS

1. Preheat the oven to 425 F.
2. In a bowl, toss everything with olive oil and salt. Spread everything onto a prepared baking sheet
3. Bake within 8-10 minutes or until crisp, and serve!

Nutrition: Calories: 38, Carbs: 2g, Fat: 2g, Protein: 3g

Carrot and Parsnips French Fries

 Prep Time: 15 minutes   Cooking Time: 20 minutes   Servings: 2

INGREDIENTS

6 large carrots
6 large parsnips
2 tbsp extra virgin olive oil
½ tsp sea salt

DIRECTIONS

1. Chop the carrots and parsnips into 2-inch sections and then cut each section into thin sticks.
2. Toss together the carrots and parsnip sticks with extra virgin olive oil and salt in a bowl and spread into a baking sheet lined with parchment paper.
3. Bake the sticks at 425 F for about 20 minutes or until browned. Serve and enjoy!

Nutrition: Calories: 209; Fat: 5 g; Carbs: 21.2 g; Protein: 1.8 g

---

Roasted Chickpeas

 Prep Time: 5 minutes   Cooking Time: 30 minutes   Servings: 2

INGREDIENTS

1 (15-oz) can of chickpeas, drained & rinsed
½ tsp olive oil
2 tsp of your favorite herbs or spice blend
¼ tsp salt

DIRECTIONS

1. Preheat the oven to 400 F.
2. In your colander, drain and rinse the chickpeas with cold water.
3. Cover a rimmed baking sheet with paper towels, place the chickpeas on it in an even layer, and blot with more paper towels until most of the liquid is absorbed.
4. Gently toss the chickpeas and olive oil in a medium bowl until combined. Sprinkle the mixture with the herbs and salt and toss again.
5. Place the chickpeas back on the baking sheet and spread in an even layer. Bake for 30 to 40 minutes, until crunchy and golden brown. Stir halfway through and serve.

Nutrition: Calories: 175; Fat: 3g; Carbs: 29g; Protein: 11g

Crispy Kale Chips

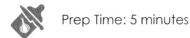 Prep Time: 5 minutes   Cooking Time: 10 minutes   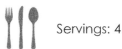 Servings: 4

INGREDIENTS

2 heads curly leaf
kale
2 tbsp olive oil

DIRECTIONS

1. Warm the oven to 325 F. Tear the kale into small pieces, removing any tough stems. Place it in a medium bowl and add the olive oil.
2. Massage the olive oil onto the kale with your hands. When kale is glossy, lay it on a baking sheet in a single layer.
3. Bake within 10 to 15 minutes until crispy. Store in an airtight container or serve immediately.

Nutrition: Calories: 70, Fat: 7.1g, Carbs: 2g, Protein: 0.8g

Stovetop Popcorn

 Prep Time: 10 minutes   Cooking Time: 5 minutes   Servings: 4

INGREDIENTS

2 tbsp olive oil
1/8 tsp salt
½ cup popcorn kernels

DIRECTIONS

1. Put the oil in the pot, and pour the corn kernels into the single layer.
2. Lower the heat and sauté with a cover top for 5 minutes. Once the popping comes, remove the heat and sprinkle the salt over it. Serve and enjoy!

Nutrition: Calories: 90, Fat: 7g, Carbs: 6g, Protein: 1g

Mixed Seed Crackers

 Prep Time: 10 minutes　　 Cooking Time: 60 minutes　　 Servings: 5

INGREDIENTS

1/4 cup amaranth
1/4 cup flaxseeds
1 tbsp sesame seeds
2 tbsp black chia seeds
1/2 cup sunflower seeds
1/4 cup pepitas
3/4 cup warm water
1 tsp sea salt

DIRECTIONS

1. In a bowl, mix amaranth, seeds, and pepitas; add warm water and sit until all water is absorbed. Stir in salt and pepper.
2. Meanwhile, preheat your oven to 320 F and line a baking tray with paper.
3. Spread the amaranth mixture onto the tray and bake in the oven for about 1 hour or until golden and crispy. Cut into 20 bars and serve.

Nutrition: Calories: 255; Fat: 4.4 g; Carbs: 2.6 g; Protein: 2.5 g

---

Trail Mix Snacks

 Prep Time: 10 minutes　　 Cooking Time: 0 minutes　　 Servings: 5

INGREDIENTS

¼ cup unsalted roasted peanuts
¼ cup whole shelled almonds
¼ cup chopped pitted dates
¼ cup dried cranberries
2 oz dried apricots

DIRECTIONS

1. In your medium bowl, mix all the ingredients until well mixed.
2. Serve and enjoy!

Nutrition:

Ginger Tahini Dip with Assorted Veggies

 Prep Time: 10 minutes   Cooking Time: 0 minutes   Servings: 8

INGREDIENTS

½ cup tahini
1 tsp grated garlic
2 tsp ground turmeric
1 tbsp grated fresh ginger
¼ cup apple cider vinegar
¼ cup water
½ tsp salt
Assorted veggie sticks, as you like

DIRECTIONS

1. Whisk tahini, turmeric, ginger, water, vinegar, garlic, and salt in a bowl until mixed well.
2. Serve with assorted veggie sticks.

Nutrition: Calories: 92; Fat: 8 g; Carbs: 4 g; Protein: 3 g

Potato Chips

 Prep Time: 5 minutes   Cooking Time: 8-10 minutes   Servings: 2

INGREDIENTS

1 lb. potatoes
2 tbsp olive oil
1 tbsp salt

DIRECTIONS

1. Preheat the oven to 425 F.
2. In a bowl, toss everything with olive oil and seasoning.
3. Spread everything onto a prepared baking sheet. Bake for 8-10 minutes or until crisp. Serve and enjoy!

Nutrition: Calories: 150, Carbs: 16g, Fat: 9g, Protein: 2g

Mango Trail Mix

 Prep Time: 5 minutes   Cooking Time: 0 minutes   Servings: 1

INGREDIENTS

2 tbsp chopped toasted cashews
2 tbsp chopped toasted Brazil nuts
2 tbsp toasted peanuts
¼ cup dried mango
2 tbsp toasted coconut flakes
1 tsp cinnamon
1 tsp cumin

DIRECTIONS

1. Mix all the fixings in your large bowl until well combined.
2. Serve and enjoy!

Nutrition: Calories: 110, Fat: 2g, Carbs: 24g, Protein: 1g

Sweet Potato Snack Bowl

 Prep Time: 10 minutes   Cooking Time: 60 minutes   Servings: 1

INGREDIENTS

1 medium sweet potato, scrubbed, poked with a fork
½ tsp cinnamon
2 tbsp chopped toasted walnuts
2 tbsp toasted pumpkin seeds

DIRECTIONS

1. Warm your oven to 350 F. Arrange the sweet potato on a paper-lined baking sheet and bake for 60 minutes or until tender; let cool and then mash together with cinnamon.
2. Transfer the mashed potatoes to a serving bowl and serve topped with chopped toasted walnuts and pumpkin seeds.

Nutrition: Calories: 297; Fat: 11 g; Carbs: 44 g; Protein: 6.7 g

Avocado Fries

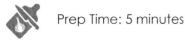 Prep Time: 5 minutes   Cooking Time: 10 minutes   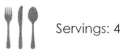 Servings: 4

INGREDIENTS

1 avocado, peeled, pitted, & cut into wedges
1 tbsp avocado oil
1 tbsp lime juice
1 tsp coriander, ground

DIRECTIONS

1. Spread the avocado wedges on a lined baking sheet, add the oil and the other ingredients, toss, and bake at 300 F for 10 minutes.
2. Divide into 2 cups and serve as a snack.

Nutrition: Calories: 236, Fat: 8.6 g, Carbs: 6.3 g, Protein: 1.9 g

---

Lemony Bean Dip with Pita Triangles

 Prep Time: 15 minutes   Cooking Time: 10 minutes   Servings: 2-3

INGREDIENTS

3 whole-wheat pita pockets, cut into eighths
Nonstick cooking spray
1 (15-oz) can of cannellini beans, drained
1 garlic clove
2 tbsp crumbled non-fat or low-fat feta
2 tsp avocado oil
1 lemon
1 tbsp chopped parsley, for garnish

DIRECTIONS

1. Preheat the oven to 400 F.
2. Arrange your pita pieces on the baking sheet and spray them on both sides with cooking spray. Bake within 10 minutes until lightly toasted. Remove from the oven and set aside.
3. Add the beans, garlic, feta, plus oil to your food processor. Grate 1/4 tsp lemon zest from your whole lemon into your processor.
4. Slice your lemon in half, then squeeze in the juice from one half. Cut your remaining lemon half into two quarters.
5. Reserving a quarter for garnish, squeeze the rest of the lemon juice into the processor. Pulse until the mixture is smooth.
6. Transfer the dip to your small bowl, garnish with the lemon wedge and parsley, and serve with the pita chips.

Nutrition: Calories: 354; Fat: 8g; Carbs: 56g; Protein: 17g

Desserts

Watermelon Popsicles

 Prep Time: 10 minutes   Cooking Time: 0 minutes   Servings: 6

INGREDIENTS

½ watermelon, seeds removed
1/3 cup honey
2 ½ cups water

DIRECTIONS

1. Mix all the ingredients and strain to remove the fiber and the form.
2. Transfer to a popsicle mold and freeze for at least 3 hours. Serve and enjoy!

Nutrition: Calories: 73; Fat: 0 g; Carbs: 14.3 g; Protein: 0.5 g

Almond-Apricot Crisp

 Prep Time: 10 minutes   Cooking Time: 25 minutes   Servings: 6

INGREDIENTS

1 tsp olive oil
1 lb. apricots
½ cup almonds, chopped
1 tbsp rolled oats
1 tsp anise seeds
2 tbsp honey

DIRECTIONS

1. Set the oven temperature to 350 F.
2. Brush olive oil in a nine-inch glass pie dish. Slice the apricots into halves and remove the pits. Put them into a pie dish.
3. Chop the almonds and sprinkle them over the apricots with anise seeds and oats on top with a drizzle of honey.
4. Bake till the topping is golden and apricots are bubbly hot within 25 minutes. Serve warm.

Nutrition: Calories: 170, Carbs: 21g, Fat: 11g, Protein: 4g

Banana Mousse

 Prep Time: 5 minutes   Cooking Time: 0 minutes   Servings: 4

INGREDIENTS

8 sliced bananas
1 medium banana
8 drops of liquid stevia
1 cup plain nonfat or low-fat yogurt
1 tsp vanilla
2 tbsp nonfat or low-fat milk

DIRECTIONS

1. Add banana, milk, stevia, and vanilla to a blender and blend them until smooth. Transfer the mixture into the bowl and add yogurt. Let it cool.
2. Transfer into your dishes and decorate with two banana slices.

Nutrition: Calories: 94, Fat: 1 g, Protein: 1 g, Carbs: 18 g

Strawberry Cheese Blintzes

 Prep Time: 5 minutes   Cooking Time: 1 minutes   Servings: 3

INGREDIENTS

1 cup nonfat or low-fat ricotta cheese
3 frozen crepes
6 fresh strawberries
2 tsp vanilla
¾ cup sugar-free orange marmalade

DIRECTIONS

1. Thaw the crepes in your refrigerator and then heat them in the microwave for 30 seconds under a damp paper towel.
2. Lay the crepes on plates, add the ricotta and sliced berries, and then roll them into a packet like a burrito.
3. Mix the vanilla and marmalade and spoon it over the tops of the crepes.

Nutrition: Calories: 274, Fat: 6.48g, Carbs: 43.71g, Protein: 10.38g

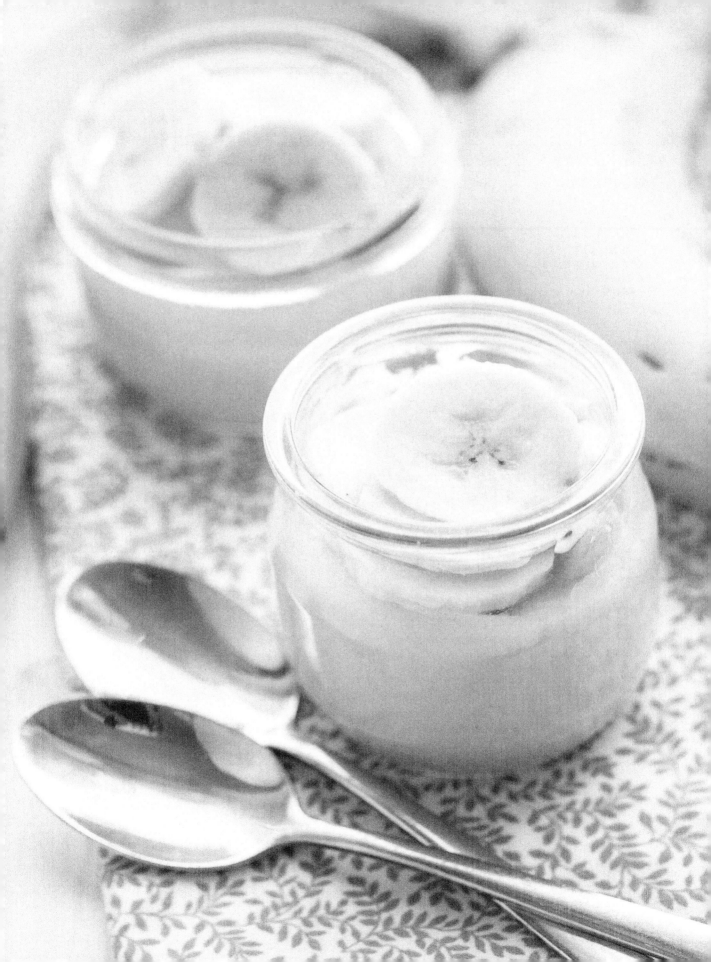

Chia Cinnamon Pudding

 Prep Time: 10 minutes   Cooking Time: 0 minutes   Servings: 6

INGREDIENTS

3 tbsp chia seed
1 packet stevia
1 cup almond milk
1/16 tsp salt
1 tsp pure vanilla extract
½ tsp. cinnamon

DIRECTIONS

1. Mix all the ingredients in a bowl.
2. Allow them to spot in the refrigerator for 2 hours. Serve and enjoy.

Nutrition: Calories: 204, Fat: 10 g, Protein: 5 g, Carbs: 21g

---

Mini Pecan Phyllo Tarts

 Prep Time: 10 minutes   Cooking Time: 15 minutes   Servings: 15 tarts

INGREDIENTS

15 mini phyllo shells
¼ tsp vanilla extract
8 drops of liquid stevia
1 tbsp olive oil
½ cup pecans
2 tbsp honey
1 large egg

DIRECTIONS

1. Allow the oven to preheat at 350 F.
2. Take a bowl and mix all the ingredients in it. Take a baking sheet and place mini pie shells in it.
3. Fill the shells with pecan mixture and bake for 15 minutes. Serve and enjoy!

Nutrition: Calories: 71, Fat: 4 g, Protein: 2 g, Carbs: 4 g

Vanilla Poached Peaches

 Prep Time: 10 minutes   Cooking Time: 30 minutes   Servings: 4

INGREDIENTS

1 cup water
1/2 tsp stevia
1 vanilla bean, split and scraped
4 large peaches, pitted and quartered
Mint leaves or ground cinnamon, for garnish

DIRECTIONS

1. Place the water, stevia, and vanilla bean into your saucepan over low heat, and stir well. Continue to simmer until the mixture thickens within 10 minutes.
2. Add the cut fruit, and poach over low heat for about 5 minutes.

Nutrition: Calories 156, Fat 0.1g, Carbs 38g, Protein 1g

Rice Pudding

 Prep Time: 10 minutes   Cooking Time: 45 minutes   Servings: 5

INGREDIENTS

½ tsp salt
3 cup semi-skim milk
2 sticks cinnamon
1/8 cup stevia
1 cup rice
6 cup water

DIRECTIONS

1. Take a saucepan and add water and cinnamon sticks to it. Allow it to boil. Add rice and cook for 30 minutes.
2. Add skim milk, salt, and stevia and cook for another 15 minutes. Serve and enjoy!

Nutrition: Calories: 372, Fat: 1 g, Carbs: 81 g, Protein: 10 g

Red Dragon Fruit Sorbet

 Prep Time: 10 minutes   Cooking Time: 0 minutes   Servings: 4

INGREDIENTS

½ cup maple syrup
¼ cup water
⅛ cup lime juice
1-½ cups cubed red dragon fruit

DIRECTIONS

1. Mix maple syrup, water, and lime juice in a saucepan over medium heat; cook for about 5 minutes. Remove from the heat and refrigerate for about 30 minutes.
2. Puree the red dragon fruit in a mixer or food processor.
3. Add the mashed red dragon fruit to the syrup mixture. Transfer the red dragon fruit mixture to an ice cream maker and freeze according to the manufacturer's instructions.

Nutrition: Calories: 116; Fat: 0.1g; Carbs: 30g; Protein: 0.1g

---

Almond Cookies

 Prep Time: 10 minutes   Cooking Time: 15 minutes   Servings: 4

INGREDIENTS

1 cup unsalted almonds
½ cup sugar substitute
¼ cup dried blueberries, chopped
1 tsp vanilla extract
1 tsp orange zest
3 egg whites

DIRECTIONS

1. Preheat the oven to 350 F.
2. Put the almonds in your food processor, then chop finely. Pour the almonds into a bowl and combine the sugar, dried blueberries, vanilla extract, and orange zest. Toss to mix.
3. Add the egg whites and mix until a dough forms. Place a spoonful of the dough on the paper sheet.
4. Place in your oven and bake for around 15 minutes, or until golden brown.

Nutrition: Calories: 82.7, Fat: 4.7 g, Carbs: 9.0 g, Protein: 2.6 g

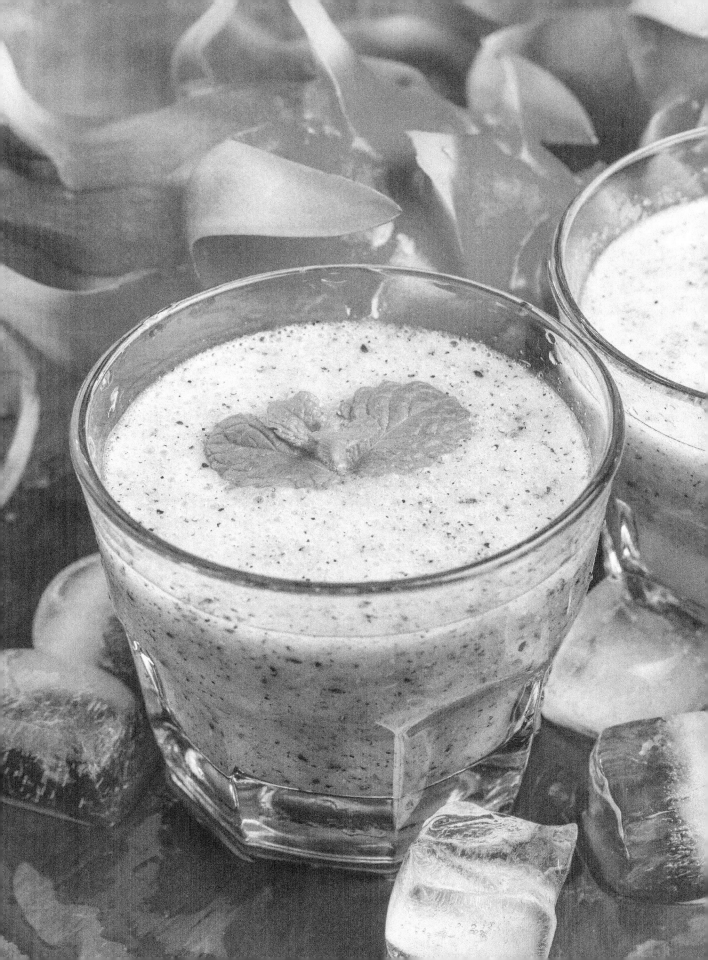

Pistachio-Stuffed Dates

 Prep Time: 10 minutes   Cooking Time: 0 minutes   Servings: 4

INGREDIENTS

½ cup unsalted pistachios shelled
¼ tsp kosher salt
8 Medjool dates, pitted

DIRECTIONS

1. In your food processor, add the pistachios and salt. Process 3-5 minutes until combined with chunky nut butter.
2. Split open the dates and spoon the pistachio nut butter into each half.

Nutrition: Calories: 220, Fat: 7g, Carbs: 41g, Protein: 4g

Strawberry Mint Yogurt

 Prep Time: 10 minutes   Cooking Time: 0 minutes   Servings: 4

INGREDIENTS

2 cups nonfat or low-fat plain yogurt
1 tbsp organic honey
2 cups strawberries, chopped
2 tbsp balsamic vinegar
2 tbsp mint leaves, finely chopped

DIRECTIONS

1. Add together the plain yogurt and organic honey in your small mixing bowl, and mix to combine.
2. In another small mixing bowl, add the chopped strawberries and balsamic vinegar. Use a fork to roughly mash the strawberries in the vinegar, then allow them to rest.
3. Divide the yogurt mixture into serving bowls, and top each with ½ cup of the strawberry mixture and ½ tbsp chopped fresh mint. Serve cold.

Nutrition: Calories: 127; Fat: 2g; Carbs: 21g; Protein: 7g

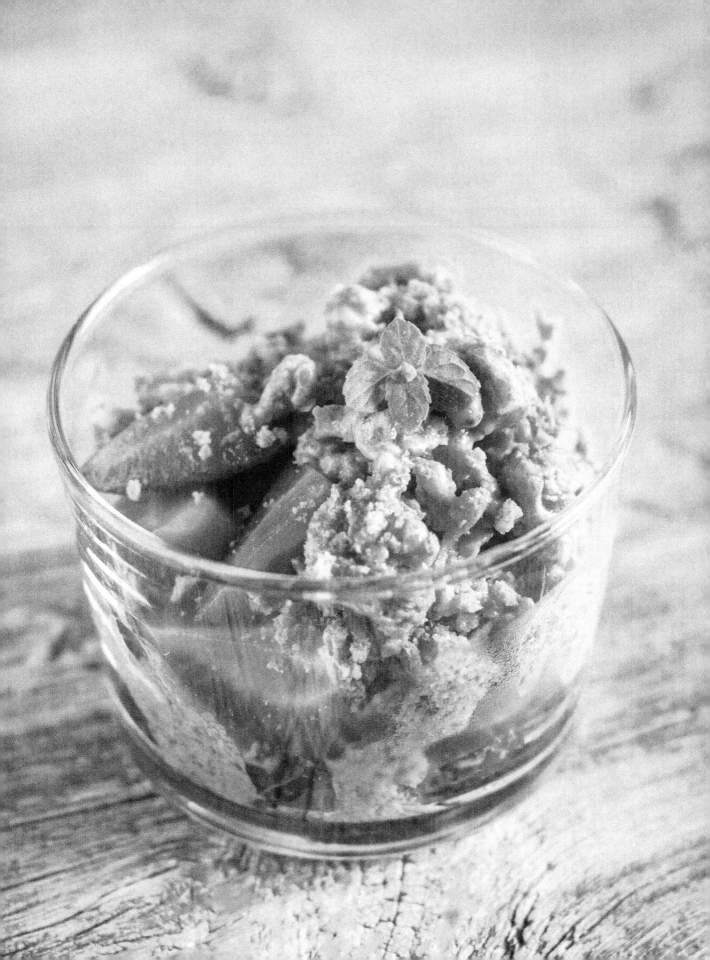

Pear Trifle

 Prep Time: 10 minutes   Cooking Time: 5 minutes   Servings: 2

INGREDIENTS

1 (14.5-oz) can of juice-packed sliced pears, drained
¼ tsp nutmeg
1 cup almond milk
1 egg yolk
½ tsp stevia
2 tbsp half-and-half
1 tab tbsp cornstarch
¼ tsp pure vanilla extract
4 fresh mint leaves (optional)

DIRECTIONS

1. Mix the pears with the nutmeg in your small bowl and set aside.
2. Stir together the milk, egg yolk, stevia, and half-and-half over medium heat in your small saucepan.
3. Quickly whisk in your cornstarch and constantly stir within 1 minute. Add your vanilla and stir until the mixture bubble, then adjust the heat to low.
4. Continue cooking until your custard is slightly thickened, within 4 to 5 minutes more. Remove the saucepan and chill the custard in your refrigerator within 30 minutes.
5. Spoon some of your custard into two small dessert dishes or parfait glasses.
6. Add a quarter of your sliced pears to each portion. Spoon more custard onto the pears and repeat until all pears and custard are used. Garnish with fresh mint (if using) and serve.

Nutrition: Calories: 203; Fat: 4g; Carbs: 37g; Protein: 6g

Broiled Mango

 Prep Time: 5 minutes   Cooking Time: 10 minutes   Servings: 2

INGREDIENTS

1 mango, peeled, seeded, and sliced
1 lime, cut into wedges

DIRECTIONS

1. Position your rack in the upper third of the oven and preheat the broiler. Line a broiler pan with aluminum foil.
2. Arrange your mango slices in a single layer in the prepared pan—broil for 8 to 10 minutes, or until browned in spots.
3. Transfer to two plates, squeeze lime wedges over the broiled mango and serve.

Nutrition: Calories: 101; Fats: 1g; Carbs: 25g; Protein: 1g

Papaya and Mint Sorbet

 Prep Time: 10 minutes

 Cooking Time: 0 minutes

 Servings: 8

INGREDIENTS

1 papaya - peeled, cored, and cut into chunks
¼ cup coconut sugar
¼ cup pineapple juice
1/8 cup mint leaves

DIRECTIONS

1. Mix the papaya, coconut sugar, pineapple juice, and mint in a mixer until smooth. Chill for 1 hour in the refrigerator.
2. Place the mixture in an ice maker and mix it according to the manufacturer's instructions. Store in an airtight container and freeze for 8 hours or overnight.

Nutrition: Calories: 25; Fat: 0.1g; Carbs: 6g; Protein: 0.3g

Pumpkin Custard

 Prep Time: 10 minutes

 Cooking Time: 35 minutes

 Servings: 4

INGREDIENTS

Nonstick cooking spray
1 cup canned pumpkin purée
½ cup nonfat or low-fat milk
1 large egg
2 tbsp maple syrup
1 tsp ground pumpkin pie spice
¼ tsp avocado oil
2 tbsp chopped pecans or walnuts

DIRECTIONS

1. Warm the oven to 350 F. Spray 4 (4-oz) ramekins with cooking spray.
2. Mix the pumpkin, milk, and egg until blended in your medium bowl. Add the syrup plus pumpkin pie spice and mix until combined.
3. Heat the oil in your small skillet over medium heat and add the nuts. Toast the nuts within 1 to 2 minutes, stirring constantly. Remove the nuts from the heat.
4. Evenly divide the pumpkin mixture between your ramekins. Top with your toasted nuts. Place the ramekins in a 9-by-11-inch baking dish.
5. Add half an inch of water to your dish and bake for 25 to 30 minutes, until firm.
6. Remove the custards from the oven, allow them to cool slightly at room temperature, and serve them warm.

Nutrition: Calories: 112; Fat: 5g; Carbs: 14g; Protein: 4g

Peach And Blueberry Tart

 Prep Time: 10 minutes   Cooking Time: 30 minutes   Servings: 6-8

INGREDIENTS

1 sheet frozen puff pastry
1 cup fresh blueberries
4 peaches, pitted and sliced
¾ tsp stevia
2 tbsp cornstarch
1 tbsp freshly squeezed lemon juice
Cooking spray
1 tbsp nonfat or low-fat milk

DIRECTIONS

1. Thaw puff pastry at room temperature within 30 minutes.
2. Preheat the oven to 400 F.
3. Toss the blueberries, peaches, stevia, cornstarch, and lemon juice in your large bowl.
4. Spray a round pie pan with your cooking spray. Unfold the pastry and place it on the prepared pie pan.
5. Arrange the peach slices, so they are slightly overlapping. Spread the blueberries on top of the peaches.
6. Drape pastry over the outside of the fruit and press pleats firmly together. Brush with milk.
7. Bake in the bottom third of your oven until the crust is golden, about 30 minutes. Cool on a rack and serve.

Nutrition: Calories: 119; Fat: 3g; Carbs: 23g; Protein: 1g

No-Oil Carrot Raisin Muffins

 Prep Time: 10 minutes   Cooking Time: 20 minutes   Servings: 10 muffins

INGREDIENTS

½ cup raisins
¼ cup molasses
1 ½ cup whole-wheat flour
½ cup skim milk
2 tsp baking powder
1/8 tsp stevia
1/3 cup shredded carrots
2 egg whites

DIRECTIONS

1. Allow the oven to preheat at 400 F.
2. Take a bowl and mix milk and carrots with egg whites. Combine flour, molasses, stevia, baking powder, and raisins. Mix well.
3. Take muffin tins and place paper liners in them. Pour batter into the tins and bake for 20 minutes. Serve and enjoy!

Nutrition: Calories: 140, Fat: 0 g, Protein: 4 g, Carbs: 32 g

Mini Fruit Pizzas with Pears

 Prep Time: 10 minutes   Cooking Time: 0 minutes   Servings: 4

INGREDIENTS

1 pear, sliced crosswise into 4 slices (¼ inch thick), seeds removed
4 tbsp peanut butter
2 tsp chopped salted roasted almonds
2 tsp maple syrup
A few non-dairy crackers

DIRECTIONS

1. Brush each pears slice with 1 tbsp of peanut butter. Lay on top of the cracker.
2. Garnish with ½ tsp of almonds and ½ tsp of maple syrup.

Nutrition: Calories: 154; Fat: 9.7g; Carbs: 14.4g; Protein: 4.6g

---

Grilled Peaches with Yogurt Drizzle

 Prep Time: 10 minutes   Cooking Time: 0 minutes   Servings: 4

INGREDIENTS

¼ cup sliced almonds
1 ½ cups plain, fat-free yogurt
2 tbsp. honey
2 tsp vanilla extract
4 ripe peaches

DIRECTIONS

1. Take a large bowl and add honey, peaches, and vanilla. Set aside for 15 minutes.
2. In another bowl, add vanilla, yogurt, and honey. Mix well and set aside.
3. Set the grill—transfer peaches to the grill and grill for four minutes.
4. In the meantime, take a small pan and add almonds to it—Cook for 3 minutes on low flame.
5. Transfer peaches to the bowl. Add yogurt and roasted almonds on the top. Serve and enjoy!

Nutrition: Calories: 191, Fat: 4 g, Carbs: 34 g, Protein: 8 g

Blueberry Ice Cream

 Prep Time: 10 minutes   Cooking Time: 45 minutes   Servings: 4

INGREDIENTS

½ lb. frozen blueber-
ries
½ cup nonfat or low-
fat sour cream
1/8 cup honey
¼ tsp vanilla extract
Blueberries for garnish

DIRECTIONS

1. Finely chop ¼ frozen blueberries with the blade of a knife. Transfer the berries to a metal bowl.
2. In a food processor, chop the remaining ¾ of frozen blueberries, add sour cream, honey, and vanilla and mix until smooth.
3. Transfer to a bowl with the chopped blueberries. Stir until everything is well mixed.
4. Cover and freeze for about 1 hour. Garnish with fresh blueberries.

Nutrition: Calories: 127; Fat: 6.2g; Carbs: 18.2g; Protein: 1.4g

---

Almond Barley Pudding

 Prep Time: 10 minutes   Cooking Time: 25 minutes   Servings: 8

INGREDIENTS

2 cups almond milk
1 cup barley
½ cup raisins
½ cup honey
2-3 tsp freshly grated
lemon zest
1 tsp vanilla extract
Pinch salt
Ground cinnamon for
dusting (optional)

DIRECTIONS

1. Mix almond milk, barley, raisins, and honey in a medium heavy sauce-pan. Bring to a boil while stirring.
2. Lower the heat and simmer, uncovered, while frequently stirring until the barley is tender and the pudding is creamy within 20 to 25 minutes.
3. Stir almost constantly towards the end to avoid burns. Add the lemon zest, vanilla, and salt and pour the pudding into a bowl or individual bowls. Let cool slightly.
4. Sprinkle with some cinnamon if desired before serving.

Nutrition: Calories: 173, Carbs: 25g, Fat: 8g, Protein: 3g

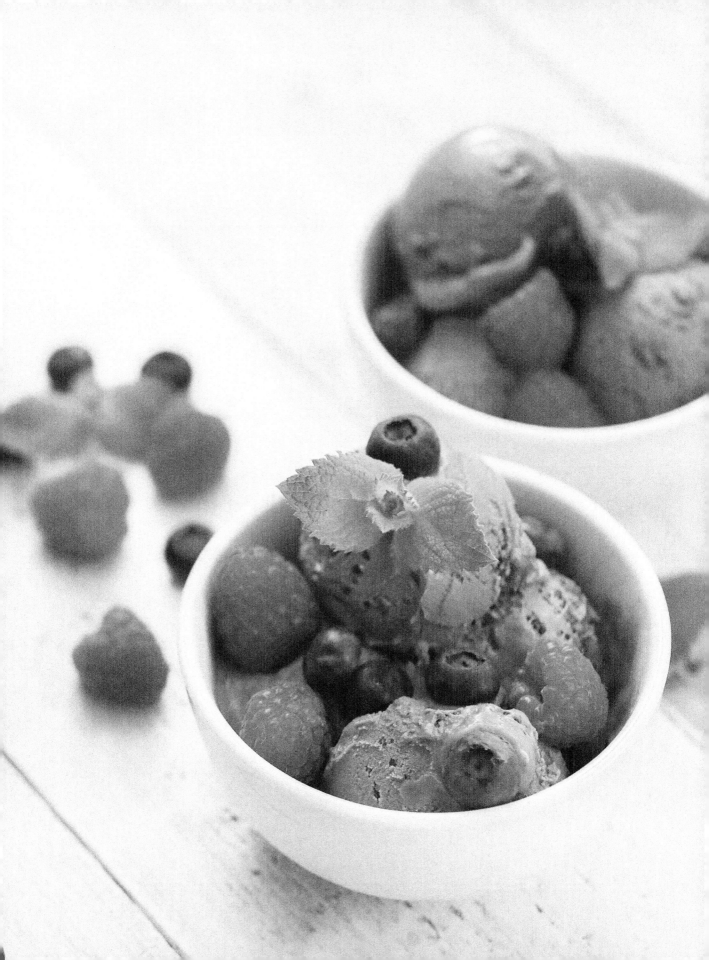

Fruit Skewers

 Prep Time: 10 minutes   Cooking Time: 0 minutes   Servings: 10

INGREDIENTS

5 strawberries, halved
1 1/2 cantaloupe, cubed
2 bananas, cut into chunks
1 apple, cored and cut into chunks

DIRECTIONS

1. Thread strawberry, cantaloupe, bananas, and apple chunks alternately onto skewers.
2. Serve them cold.

Nutrition: Calories: 76, Fat: 1 g, Carbs: 10 g, Protein: 2 g

Peanut Rice Crisp Bars

 Prep Time: 15 minutes   Cooking Time: 0 minutes   Servings: 8 bars

INGREDIENTS

2 cups crisp rice cereal
¼ cup honey
¼ cup crunchy peanut butter

DIRECTIONS

1. Line your 9-by-5-inch loaf pan with parchment paper.
2. Put the cereal in a medium bowl.
3. Put the honey and peanut butter in a small microwave-safe bowl. Heat within 30 seconds in the microwave on high.
4. Remove and stir the mixture, then microwave it for 30 more seconds at 50 percent power. Pour the honey mixture over your cereal and stir to combine.
5. Transfer the cereal mixture to the loaf pan, pressing it into the bottom.
6. Set your pan aside at room temperature to cool. When the mixture has cooled, cut it into 8 equal bars.

Nutrition: Calories: 94; Fat: 4g; Carbs: 14g; Protein: 2g

Strawberry Bruschetta

 Prep Time: 15 minutes

 Cooking Time: 0 minutes

 Servings: 12

INGREDIENTS

1 loaf of sliced Ciabatta bread
8 oz nonfat or low-fat goat cheese
1 cup basil leaves
2 containers of strawberries, sliced
5 tbsp balsamic glaze

DIRECTIONS

1. Wash and slice strawberries; set aside. Wash and chop the basil leaves; set aside.
2. Slice the ciabatta bread and spread some goat cheese evenly on each slice; add strawberries, balsamic glaze, and top with basil leaves. Serve on a platter.

Nutrition: Calories 80, Fats 2 g, Carbs 12 g, Proteins 3 g

Grilled Apricots with Cinnamon

 Prep Time: 5 minutes

 Cooking Time: 10 minutes

 Servings: 4

INGREDIENTS

4 large apricots, halved and pitted
1 tbsp extra-virgin olive oil
1/4 tsp ground cinnamon

DIRECTIONS

1. Brush with oil on both sides of each apricot half, and put flat
2. On the hot grill or grill pan, side down. Grill for around 4 minutes, turn over the apricot halves, and grill until soft for a few more minutes.
3. Sprinkle with cinnamon and cut the apricots from the grill. Enjoy being wet or cold.

Nutrition: Calories: 245, Fat: 7g, Carbs:6g, Protein: 20g

Lemon Cookies

 Prep Time: 15 minutes

 Cooking Time: 10 minutes

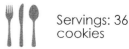 Servings: 36 cookies

INGREDIENTS

2 1/2 cups white whole-wheat flour
¾ tsp stevia
1 tbsp sodium-free baking powder
3/4 cup olive oil
2 large lemons, juice, and grated zest
1 tbsp pure vanilla extract

DIRECTIONS

1. Warm the oven to 350 F. Mix the flour, stevia, plus baking powder into a mixing bowl. Put the rest of the fixing and stir to form a stiff dough.
2. Drop by rounded tablespoons onto an ungreased baking sheet—Bake within 10 minutes.
3. Remove, and let it cool on the sheet for a few minutes before transferring it to a wire rack to cool fully. Serve immediately.

Nutrition: Calories: 106, Fat: 5 g, Carbs: 15 g, Protein: 1 g

Roasted Pineapple with Maple Glaze

 Prep Time: 10 minutes

 Cooking Time: 20 minutes

 Servings: 4

INGREDIENTS

1 ripe pineapple
Olive oil cooking spray
1/4 cup pure maple syrup

DIRECTIONS

1. Preheat the oven to 425 F.
2. Cut the pineapple lengthwise into quarters using a big, sharp knife. To yield 8 wedges, cut each quarter lengthwise. For another use, reserve 4 of the wedges.
3. Use your paring knife to cut the flesh from the rind into one piece while dealing with 1 pineapple wedge at a time.
4. Break the flesh into 5 large chunks vertically, holding them nestled in the rind.
5. Arrange the pineapple wedges in a baking dish and brush lightly with oil. Roast for about 15 minutes before it just begins to brown.
6. Brush the maple syrup over the pineapple and bake for about 5 more minutes until the pineapple is glazed.
7. Transfer to four large plates, drizzle with the baking dish liquid, and serve warm.

Nutrition: Calories: 290, Fat: 6g, Carbohydrates: 17g, Protein:10g

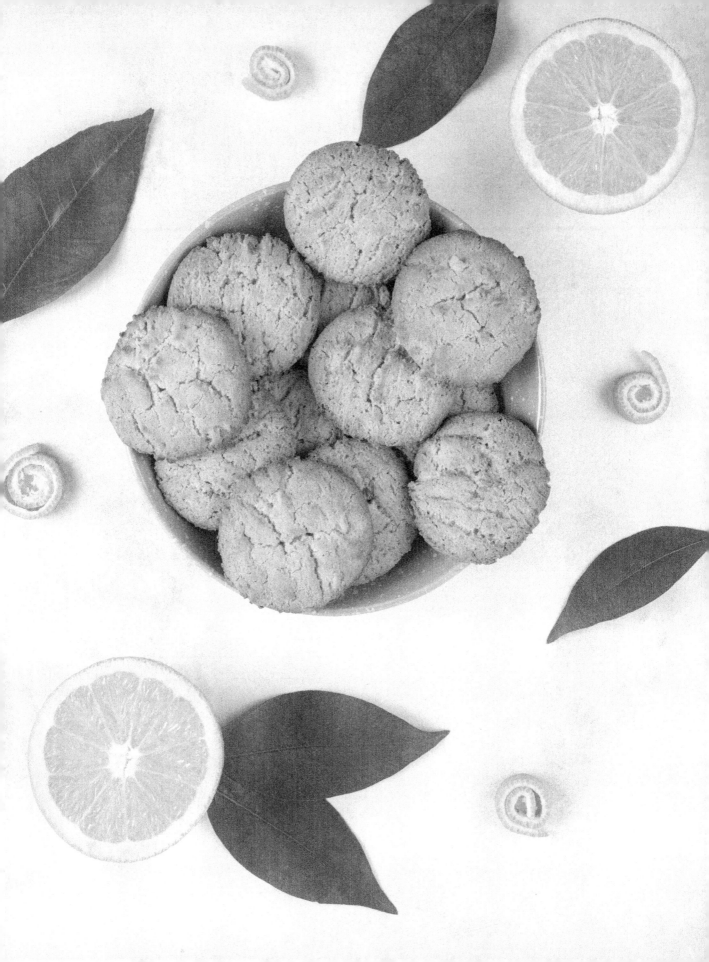

Grapefruit Compote

 Prep Time: 5 minutes   Cooking Time: 8 minutes   Servings: 4

INGREDIENTS

1 cup palm sugar
64 oz sugar-free red grapefruit juice
1/2 cup chopped mint
2 peeled and cubed grapefruits

DIRECTIONS

1. Combine all the fixings into your pot.
2. Cook on low for 8 minutes, then divide into bowls and serve!

Nutrition: Calories: 131, Fat 4g, Carbs 12g, Protein 2g

Kiwi Bars

 Prep Time: 20 minutes   Cooking Time: 0 minutes   Servings: 4

INGREDIENTS

1 cup olive oil
1 1/2 bananas, peeled and chopped
1/3 cup coconut sugar
1/4 cup lemon juice
1 tsp lemon zest, grated
3 kiwis, peeled and chopped

DIRECTIONS

1. Mix bananas with kiwis, almost all the oil, sugar, lemon juice, and lemon zest in your food processor, and pulse well.
2. Grease a pan with the remaining oil, pour the kiwi mix, spread, keep in the fridge for 30 minutes, slice, and serve.

Nutrition: Calories 206, Fat 4g, Carbs 20g, Protein 10g

Smoothies & Drinks

Blueberry Smoothie

 Prep Time: 5 minutes   Cooking Time: 0 minutes   Servings: 2

INGREDIENTS

½ cup frozen blueberries
1 cup unsweetened almond milk
1 tbsp almond butter
¼ cup ice cubes
1 pinch of salt

DIRECTIONS

1. Mix all of the fixings in your blender and blend until smooth.
2. Serve and enjoy.

Nutrition: Calories: 170, Carbs: 41g, Fat: 0g, Protein: 1g

Fresh Berry Mint Infused Water

 Prep Time: 5 minutes   Cooking Time: 0 minutes   Servings: 8

INGREDIENTS

½ cup strawberries
½ cup blackberries
3 mint sprigs
8 cups water

DIRECTIONS

1. Mix the water, strawberries, blackberries, and mint in a large pitcher.
2. Before drinking, cover the infused water and chill for at least 1 hour.

Nutrition: Calories: 7, Fat: 0g, Carbs: 2g, Protein: 0g

Fizzy Lemon and Strawberry Punch

 Prep Time: 10 minutes   Cooking Time: 0 minutes   Servings: 12

INGREDIENTS

1 cup honey
10 strawberries
2 cups freshly squee-
zed lemon juice
7 cups of water

DIRECTIONS

1. Mix all the ingredients; you can divide the ingredients into two or three if your mixer is not big enough.
2. Chill in the fridge and serve cold.

Nutrition: Calories: 141; Fat: 0.3 g; Carbs: 30.5 g; Protein: 1.1 g

---

Watermelon Smoothie

 Prep Time: 5 minutes   Cooking Time: 0 minutes   Servings: 1

INGREDIENTS

2 cups watermelon
1 cup almond milk
1 cup nonfat or low-
fat vanilla yogurt
2 tbsp maple syrup
1 cup ice

DIRECTIONS

1. In a blender, place all ingredients and blend until smooth.
2. Pour the smoothie into a glass and serve.

Nutrition: Calories: 75, Carbs: 19g, Fat: 0g, Protein: 2g

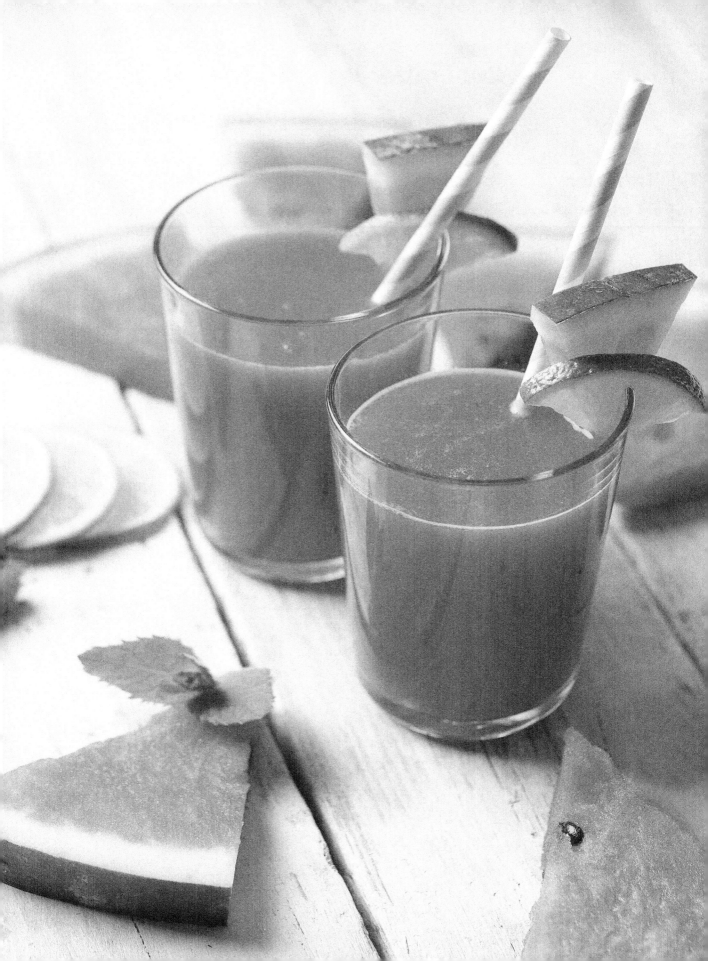

Cucumber-Watermelon Juice

 Prep Time: 5 minutes   Cooking Time: 0 minutes   Servings: 4

INGREDIENTS

5 cups chopped see-
dless watermelon
1 cup chopped un-
peeled cucumber
10 fresh mint leaves
Juice of ½ lime

DIRECTIONS

1. Blend the watermelon and cucumber in the blender and blend high until smooth.
2. Add the mint and lime juice to the last blend. Serve chilled.

Nutrition: Calories: 66, Fat: 0.9g, Carbs: 15g, Protein: 2g

Pear and Mango Smoothie

 Prep Time: 5 minutes   Cooking Time: 0 minutes   Servings: 1

INGREDIENTS

1 ripe mango, cored
and chopped
½ mango, peeled,
pitted, and chopped
1 cup kale, chopped
½ cup nonfat or low-
fat plain Greek yogurt
2 ice cubes

DIRECTIONS

1. Add pear, mango, yogurt, kale, and mango to a blender and puree.
2. Put the ice and blend until you have a smooth texture. Serve and enjoy!

Nutrition: Calories: 293, Fat: 8g, Carbs: 53g, Protein: 8g

Pineapple Smoothie

 Prep Time: 5 minutes   Cooking Time: 0 minutes   Servings: 1

INGREDIENTS

½ cup fresh or drained
canned pineapple
1/8 cup orange juice
¼ cup nonfat or low-fat
plain yogurt
1/8 cup water
2 ice cubes, crushed

DIRECTIONS

1. Combine pineapple, orange juice, plain yogurt, water, and ice cubes in a blender.
2. Cover and blend until smooth.

Nutrition: Calories: 99; Fat: 0.9g; Carbs: 18.4g; Protein: 4.1g

---

Mango Ginger Smoothie

 Prep Time: 5 minutes   Cooking Time: 0 minutes   Servings: 2

INGREDIENTS

1 cup cooked lentils
cooled
2 cups frozen mango
chunks
1-½ cups orange juice
2 tsp chopped fresh
ginger
2 tsp maple syrup (op-
tional)
Pinch of ground
nutmeg, plus more for
garnish
6 ice cubes

DIRECTIONS

1. Put the lentils, mango, orange juice, ginger, maple syrup, nutmeg, and ice cubes in a mixer.
2. Beat over high heat for 2 to 3 minutes until smooth. Garnish with more nutmeg if desired.

Nutrition: Calories: 292; Fat: 1.4g; Carbs: 62.8g; Protein: 11.3g

Almond Butter and Blueberry Smoothie

 Prep Time: 5 minutes   Cooking Time: 0 minutes   Servings: 2

INGREDIENTS

1 cup almond milk
1 cup blueberries
4 ice cubes
1 scoop of vanilla
protein powder
1 tbsp almond butter
1 tbsp chia seeds

DIRECTIONS

1. Use a blender to mix the almond butter, vanilla protein powder, chia seeds, almond milk, ice cubes, and blueberries until the consistency is smooth.
2. Serve and enjoy!

Nutrition: Calories: 230, Fat: 8.1 g, Carbs: 20 g, Protein: 21.6 g

---

Green Apple Smoothie

 Prep Time: 5 minutes   Cooking Time: 0 minutes   Servings: 2

INGREDIENTS

1 cup apple cider:
1 small banana
1-2 cup kale, stems
removed
pinch of cinnamon
1 cup green apple
cut into chunks
1 cup of water or ice

DIRECTIONS

1. In a blender, add all fixings and blend until smooth.
2. Serve and enjoy!

Nutrition: Calories 233, Fat 0.5g, Carbs 56.4g, Protein 2g

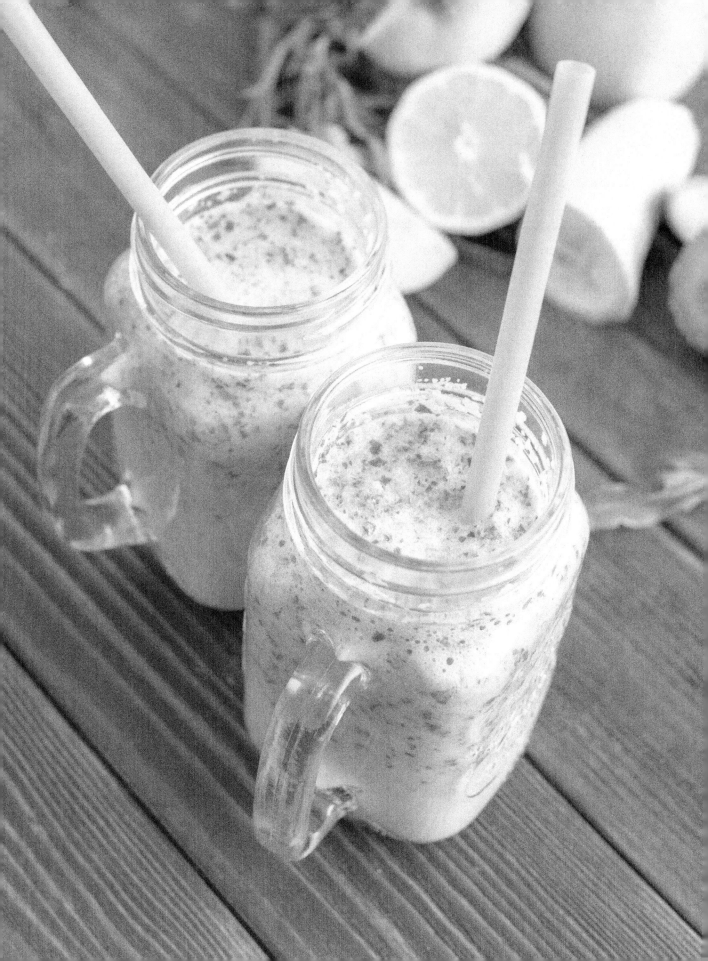

Mint and Cumin Salted Lassi

 Prep Time: 5 minutes   Cooking Time: 0 minutes   Servings: 2

INGREDIENTS

1 tsp cumin seeds
½ cup mint leaves
1 cup nonfat or
low-fat plain yogurt,
unsweetened
½ cup water

DIRECTIONS

1. Toast the cumin seeds in a dry skillet over medium heat for 1 to 2 minutes, until fragrant.
2. Transfer the seeds to your blender, then add the mint, yogurt, and water, and process until smooth. Serve immediately.

Nutrition: Calories: 114, Fat: 6g, Carbs: 5g, Protein: 10g

Kiwi Strawberry Banana Smoothie

 Prep Time: 5 minutes   Cooking Time: 0 minutes   Servings: 4

INGREDIENTS

2 cups sliced fresh
strawberries
1 small banana, sliced
6 oz nonfat or low-fat
Greek yogurt
1 cup ice cubes
½ kiwi fruit, peeled
and sliced

DIRECTIONS

1. In a mixer, mix all ingredients. Cover and mix until smooth.
2. Serve and enjoy!

Nutrition: Calories: 124, Fat: 1g, Carbs: 28g, Protein: 3g

Green Smoothie

 Prep Time: 5 minutes　　 Cooking Time: 0 minutes　　 Servings: 1

INGREDIENTS

1 avocado, sliced
1 cup spinach
1 banana, sliced
½ cup cauliflower florets
2 dates
1 cup almond milk

DIRECTIONS

1. 1. In a blender, place all ingredients and blend until smooth.
2. 2. Pour the smoothie into a glass and serve.

Nutrition: Calories: 160, Carbs: 39g, Fat: 1g, Protein: 3g

Cantaloupe Smoothie

 Prep Time: 5 minutes　　 Cooking Time: 0 minutes　　 Servings: 2

INGREDIENTS

2 ½ cups frozen cantaloupe, cubed
½ cup nonfat or low-fat milk
1 frozen banana, sliced
6 oz nonfat or low-fat vanilla Greek yogurt
½ cup ice
1 tsp honey

DIRECTIONS

1. Place the milk, banana, yogurt, ice, and honey in a blender. Work and mix the fixings till incorporated and creamy.
2. Toss in the cantaloupe pieces - process until incorporated and creamy smooth. Serve immediately.

Nutrition: Calories: 214, Fat: 1g, Carbs: 46g, Protein: 11g

Papaya Mint Infused Water

 Prep Time: 5 minutes   Cooking Time: 0 minutes   Servings: 10

INGREDIENTS

1 cup fresh papaya, peeled, seeded, and diced
2 tbsps. chopped fresh mint leaves
10 cups distilled or filtered water

DIRECTIONS

1. In a large pitcher, add the papaya and mint. Then pour in the water.
2. Stir well, and refrigerate the pitcher to infuse overnight if possible. Serve cold.

Nutrition: Calories: 2, Fat: 0g, Carbs: 0g, Fiber: 0g, Protein: 0g

---

Peach Carrot Ginger Water

 Prep Time: 5 minutes   Cooking Time: 0 minutes   Servings: 10

INGREDIENTS

2 peaches, peeled, pitted, and chopped
1 large carrot, peeled and grated
1-inch piece peeled fresh ginger, lightly crushed
3 fresh thyme sprigs
10 cups water

DIRECTIONS

1. Add the peaches, carrot, ginger, and thyme to a large pitcher. Stir in the water, and mix to combine.
2. Place the pitcher in your refrigerator and leave to infuse overnight. Serve cold.

Nutrition: Calories: 40, Fat: 0g, Carbs: 10.7g, Protein: 0.3g

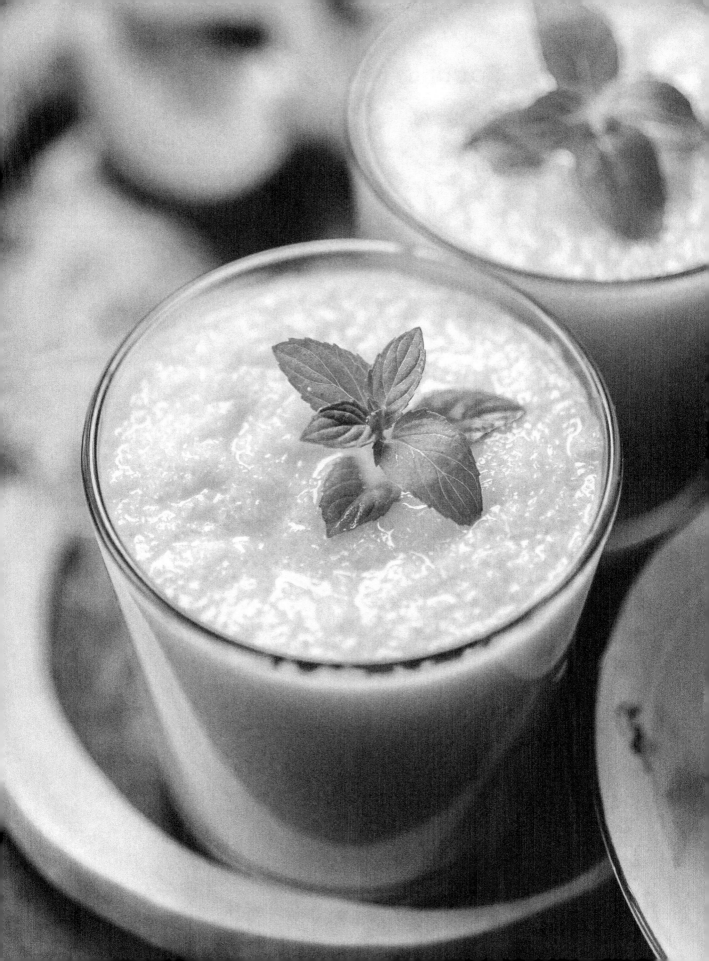

Coconut Pineapple Smoothie

 Prep Time: 5 minutes   Cooking Time: 0 minutes   Servings: 1

INGREDIENTS

2 cup pineapple
¼ cup coconut milk
1 cup pineapple juice
2 tbsp coconut flakes
½ cup nonfat or low-fat yogurt
1 tbsp honey

DIRECTIONS

1. In a blender, place all ingredients and blend until smooth.
2. Pour the smoothie into a glass and serve.

Nutrition: Calories: 200, Carbs: 33g, Fat: 7g, Protein: 3g

Rice Milk

 Prep Time: 5 minutes   Cooking Time: 5 minutes   Servings: 4

INGREDIENTS

1 cup long-grain white rice
4 cups water
½ tsp. vanilla extract (optional)

DIRECTIONS

1. Toast the rice in a medium dry skillet over medium heat for 5 minutes, until lightly browned.
2. Transfer the rice to a jar or bowl, and add the water. Cover, refrigerate and soak overnight.
3. Add the rice, water, and vanilla (if using) to a blender and process until smooth.
4. Pour the milk into your glass jar or bowl with a fine-mesh strainer. Serve immediately, or cover, refrigerate and serve within three days. Shake before using.

Nutrition: Calories: 112, Fat: 0g, Carbs: 24g, Protein: 0g

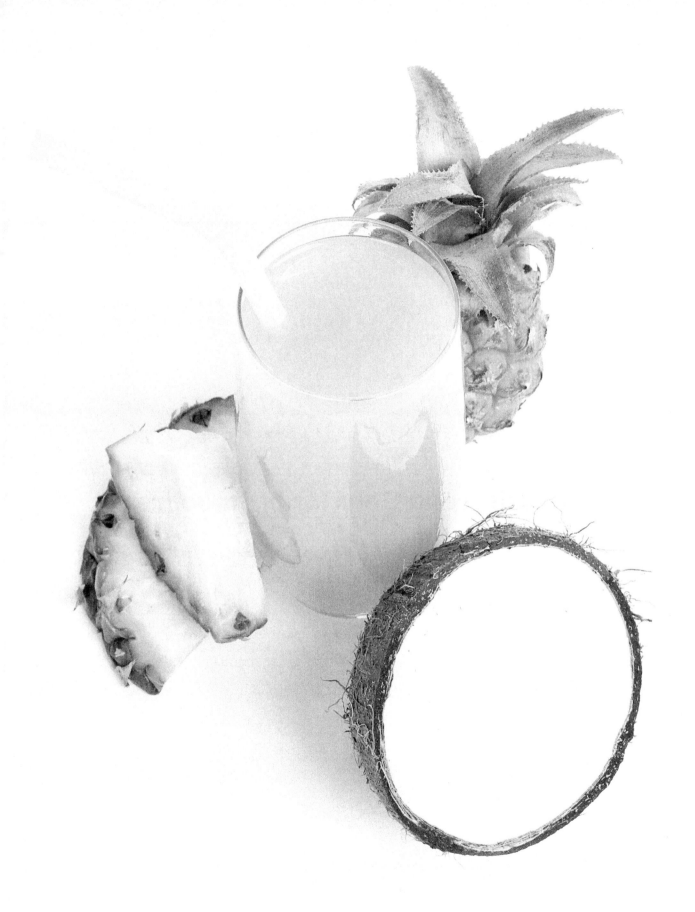

Coconut Strawberry Smoothie

 Prep Time: 5 minutes Cooking Time: 0 minutes Servings: 2

INGREDIENTS

1 tbsp shredded coconut
1/2 cup of frozen strawberries
1 cup of unsweetened almond milk
1 tsp chia seeds
2 tbsp avocado
1 tbsp low-fat cream

DIRECTIONS

1. Add all the fixings to a blender. Pulse it on high until smooth and creamy.
2. Pour in a glass and enjoy.

Nutrition: Calories: 98, Fat: 0.4 g, Carbs: 11 g, Protein: 8.2 g

---

Banana Cauliflower Smoothie

 Prep Time: 5 minutes Cooking Time: 0 minutes Servings: 1

INGREDIENTS

½ cup frozen riced cauliflower
¼ cup frozen mixed berries
½ cup sliced frozen banana
1 cup unsweetened coconut milk
1 tsp honey (optional)

DIRECTIONS

1. Combine riced cauliflower, mixed berries, banana, coconut milk, and honey in a blender.
2. Cover and blend until smooth. Serve and enjoy!

Nutrition: Calories 168, Fat 4.4g, Carbs 31.7g, Protein 2.1g

Turmeric Ginger Lemonade

 Prep Time: 5 minutes   Cooking Time: 5 minutes   Servings: 2

INGREDIENTS

2½ cups water
1 tsp ginger powder
1 tsp turmeric powder
¼ cup lemon juice
2 tsp aloe vera (optional)
2 tsp erythritol or 2 drops
of liquid stevia (optional)
¼ tsp finely ground Hima-
layan salt
Pinch of ground black
pepper
6 fresh mint leaves
1 small lemon, cut into
wedges

DIRECTIONS

1. In a medium-sized saucepan, add the water, ginger, and turmeric, and bring to a boil.
2. Remove, and stir in the lemon juice, aloe vera (if using), sweetener (if using), salt, and pepper.
3. Use a spoon to stir and let it cool for 1 hour, until completely cooled.
4. In a 24-ounce or larger airtight container, place the mixture. Add the mint leaves, squeeze in the lemon juice and drop the wedges into the lemonade. Chill in the refrigerator until cold.
5. When ready to enjoy, pour into two 12-ounce (350-ml) or larger glasses.

Nutrition: Calories: 13, Fat: 0.4g, Carbs: 1.5g, Protein: 0.4g

Peanut Butter Smoothie

 Prep Time: 5 minutes   Cooking Time: 0 minutes   Servings: 1

INGREDIENTS

2 cups banana
1 tbsp flax seeds
1 cup almond milk
1 tsp vanilla extract
2 tbsp peanut butter

DIRECTIONS

1. In a blender, place all ingredients and blend until smooth.
2. Pour the smoothie in a glass and serve.

Nutrition: Calories: 303, Carbs: 45g, Fat: 9g, Protein: 16g

Spinach Strawberry Smoothie

 Prep Time: 5 minutes

 Cooking Time: 0 minutes

 Servings: 1

INGREDIENTS

2 cups banana
2 cups strawberries
2 cups spinach
2 chia seeds

DIRECTIONS

1. In a blender, place all ingredients and blend until smooth.
2. Pour the smoothie into a glass and serve.

Nutrition: Calories: 255, Carbs: 52g, Fat: 3g, Protein: 12g

Pear Smoothie

 Prep Time: 5 minutes

 Cooking Time: 0 minutes

 Servings: 1

INGREDIENTS

1 pear, cored and quartered
½ fennel bulb
1 thin slice of fresh ginger
1 cup packed spinach
½ cucumber, peeled
½ cup water
Ice (optional)

DIRECTIONS

1. Add the pear, fennel, ginger, spinach, cucumber, water, and ice (if using) to a blender and blend until smooth.
2. Serve in glasses and garnish with your choices.

Nutrition: Calories: 147, Fat: 1g, Carbs: 37g, Protein: 4g

Orange Juice Smoothie

 Prep Time: 5 minutes   Cooking Time: 0 minutes   Servings: 2

INGREDIENTS

1 cup nonfat or low-fat vanilla frozen yogurt
¾ cup nonfat or low-fat milk
¼ cup no-sugar frozen orange juice

DIRECTIONS

1. Toss each of the fixings into your blender - mixing till creamy.
2. Serve in a cold mug and enjoy them right away.

Nutrition: Calories 220, Fat 1g, Carbs 41g, Protein 12g

28 Days Meal Plan

DAY	BREAKFAST	LUNCH	DINNER	SNACKS	DESSERTS
1	Buckwheat Pancakes	Chicken Tenders with Pineapple	Garlic Turkey Breasts with Lemon	Quinoa Energy Balls	Watermelon Popsicles
2	Coconut Yogurt with Acai Berry Granola	Glazed Tempeh	Seafood Fettuccine	Gingerbread Balls	Pistachio-Stuffed Dates
3	Amaranth Porridge	Grilled Turkey Teriyaki	Orange Maple Glazed Salmon	Zucchini Chips	Almond Cookies
4	Broccoli Frittata	Steamed Chicken with Mushroom & Ginger	Buckwheat with Mushrooms & Green Onions	Spinach Balls	Rice Pudding
5	Cassava Crepes	Millet Lettuce Wraps	Pasta e Fagioli	Roasted Sweet Potato Fries	Red Dragon Fruit Sorbet
6	Breakfast Overnight Oats	White Fish Fillets with Sweet Potato Flakes	Baked Mustard-Lime Chicken	Amaranth Pop Corns	Vanilla Poached Peaches
7	Greek Omelet	Cod Parcels with Mushrooms and Spinach	Red Lentil Soup with Tomato Sauce	Taro Chips	Almond-Apricot Crisp
8	Turkey Sweet Potato Breakfast Casserole	Chickpea Veggie Sauté	Cheesy Tortilla Casserole	Oat Nuggets	Mini Pecan Phyllo Tarts
9	Artichoke Pancakes	Turkey Salad	Baked Flounder with Tomatoes and Basil	Guacamole with Jicama	Chia Cinnamon Pudding
10	Eggs Baked in Mushrooms	Chicken And Rice	Chicken with Broccoli Stir-Fry	Baked Apples	Banana Mousse
11	Turmeric Oatmeal	Baked Lemon Salmon with Zucchini	Chicken and Celery Soup	Squash Chips	Strawberry Cheese Blintzes
12	Amaranth with Toasted Walnuts	Chicken Souvlaki Kebabs	All Spice-Crusty Roasted Salmon	Vegetable Chips with Rosemary Salt	Strawberry Mint Yogurt
13	Kale Frittata	Sautéed Turkey with Cabbage	Baked Halibut Steaks	Roasted Lentil Snack Mix	Fruit Skewers
14	Mixed Berries Yogurt	Buddha Bowl	Crispy Almond Chicken Breast	Cucumber Chips	Almond Barley Pudding

DAY	BREAKFAST	LUNCH	DINNER	SNACKS	DESSERTS
15	French Toast	Smashed Chickpea Salad Sandwich	Rosemary Lemon Chicken	Crispy Potato Skins	Blueberry Ice Cream
16	Rutabaga Breakfast Hash	Chicken Fajita Bowl	Almond Noodles with Cauliflower	Turmeric Cashew Nut Balls	Grilled Peaches with Yogurt Drizzle
17	Banana Pancakes	Italian Fish Fillet	Pan-Seared Chicken with Turnip Greens	Carrot and Parsnips French Fries	Pear Trifle
18	Salmon Egg Salad	Chicken and Cauliflower Rice Bowls	Minestrone	Ginger Tahini Dip with Assorted Veggies	Mini Fruit Pizzas with Pears
19	Avocado Toast with Hummus	Kale and Cottage Pasta	Sea Bass with Tomatoes, Olives, and Capers	Potato Chips	No-Oil Carrot Raisin Muffins
20	Mushroom Omelet	Ginger Glazed Tuna	Summer Ratatouille	Trail Mix Snacks	Peach And Blueberry Tart
21	Banana And Apple Pancakes	Cauliflower Shawarma with Tahini	Eggplant and Chickpea Stew	Mixed Seed Crackers	Pumpkin Custard
22	Banana Walnut Pancakes	Tuna Melt Stuffed Tomatoes	Buckwheat with Bow-Tie Pasta	Stovetop Popcorn	Broiled Mango
23	Carrot Muffins	Poached Fish in Tomato-Caper Sauce	Stewed Chicken with Asparagus and Carrot	Roasted Chickpeas	Papaya and Mint Sorbet
24	Nutmeg Apple Frozen Yogurt	Shrimp with Mushrooms	Casserole Pizza	Crispy Kale Chips	Peanut Rice Crisp Bars
25	Brown Rice Breakfast Bowl	Chicken Pizza	Sweet-and-Sour Trout with Chard	Mango Trail Mix	Kiwi Bars
26	Leek Frittata	Artichoke Heart and Chickpea–Stuffed Portabellas	Italian Herb Turkey Cutlets	Lemony Bean Dip with Pita Triangles	Grapefruit Compote
27	Orange Muffins	Chicken and Brussels Sprouts Skillet	Weeknight Fish Skillet	Avocado Fries	Roasted Pineapple with Maple Glaze
28	Barley Oats Granola with Almond	Salmon Burgers	Green Pesto Pasta	Sweet Potato Snack Bowl	Lemon Cookies

Printed in Great Britain
by Amazon

17060754R00081